D1516106

Unlocking
THE
Healing
Code

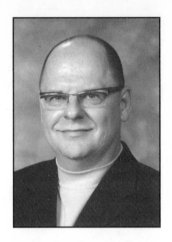

About the Author

Dr. Bruce Forciea is an instructor in anatomy and physiology at Moraine Park Technical College in Wisconsin, while continuing his part-time chiropractic practice, lecturing, and writing about healing. For more information about *Unlocking the Healing Code* please visit: www .informationalhealing.com. Here you will find a variety of support materials including a vast number of articles on alternative medicine, healing, New Age philosophy, and the principles in this book. You can also subscribe to a free newsletter, download podcasts about the book, and listen to New Age music.

Unlocking THE Healing Code

Discover the 7 Keys to Unlimited Healing Power

Dr. Bruce Forciea

Llewellyn Publications
Woodbury, Minnesota

Unlocking the Healing Code: Discover the 7 Keys to Unlimited Healing Power © 2007 by Dr. Bruce Forciea. All rights reserved. No part of this book may be used or reproduced in any manner whatsoever, including Internet usage, without written permission from Llewellyn Publications except in the case of brief quotations embodied in critical articles and reviews.

First Edition
First Printing, 2007

Book design by Donna Burch
Cover art © Hammond Nagy/Designpics.com/PunchStock
Cover design by Ellen Dahl
Editing by Connie Hill
Llewellyn is a registered trademark of Llewellyn Worldwide, Ltd.

Library of Congress Cataloging-in-Publication Data

Forciea, Bruce, 1951–
  Unlocking the healing code : discover the 7 keys to unlimited healing
power / Bruce Forciea.—1st ed.
    p. cm.
  Includes bibliographical references and index.
  ISBN 978-0-7387-1077-8
  1. Alternative medicine. 2. Healing. 3. Information theory. I. Title.
  R733.F725 2007
  613—dc22
                              2007040169

Llewellyn Worldwide does not participate in, endorse, or have any authority or responsibility concerning private business transactions between our authors and the public.

  All mail addressed to the author is forwarded but the publisher cannot, unless specifically instructed by the author, give out an address or phone number.

  Any Internet references contained in this work are current at publication time, but the publisher cannot guarantee that a specific location will continue to be maintained. Please refer to the publisher's website for links to authors' websites and other sources.

Note: The practices, techniques, and concepts described in this book should not be used as an alternative to professional medical treatment. This book does not attempt to give any medical diagnosis, treatment, prescription, or suggestion for medication in relation to any human disease, pain, injury, deformity, or physical condition.

  The author and publisher of this book are not responsible in any manner whatsoever for any injury which may occur through any concepts, instructions, or recommendations contained herein. It is recommended that before beginning any healing practice you consult with your physician to determine whether you are medically, physically, and mentally fit to undertake the practice.

Llewellyn Publications
A Division of Llewellyn Worldwide, Ltd.
2143 Wooddale Drive, Dept. 978-0-7387-1077-8
Woodbury, Minnesota 55125-2989, U.S.A.
www.llewellyn.com

Printed in the United States of America

To the memory of my mother for her inspiration
To Susan for her love
To Grace for her joy

Acknowledgments

I am grateful to the many people who have inspired and helped me through this project. First and foremost is my wife Susan who endured endless technical conversations and supported my ideas during the years of development. I also wish to thank the wonderful people at Llewellyn Worldwide for recognizing the potential buried in a roughly presented manuscript—in particular, Carrie Obry for her developmental experience and inspiration throughout the project. Special thanks to Stephanie Golden for editing the early version of the manuscript and to Lee Sauer at Moraine Park Technical College for his suggestions in the beginning stages of development. Lastly, thank you to those who shared their healing stories with me so that we all can learn from their experiences.

Contents

INTRODUCTION

Heart attack! That's what came to mind as I lay in bed one evening, heart pounding, pain in my chest, sweating, and dizzy. I was alone in Australia, ten thousand miles from home. I struggled to the phone to make a desperate call to one of the few people I knew there. I wondered if I would lose consciousness.

My friend came. The trip to the hospital seemed to take an eternity. Denial. The logical part of my brain kicked in. How could a twenty-four-year-old, in excellent health, have a heart attack?

We reached a part of Sydney I had not seen since my arrival a year earlier. The hospital was old and sterile. Oddly enough, the emergency room was vacant. Several nurses and an intern looked at me. They appeared to be my age. I was scared and hyperventilating. An electrocardiogram, blood work, and a chest x-ray were all negative. The pain, palpitations, sweating, and dizziness stopped after about two hours. It was over. No heart attack. Relief. One night in the hospital followed by a discharge and diagnosis of paroxysmal tachycardia (very fast heart rate of unknown origin).

Two weeks, and over thirty attacks later, I realized this problem wasn't going away. I had changed from a young, healthy athlete to a disabled, neurotic person living in fear. I felt condemned. I became obsessed with taking my own pulse, maybe fifty times a day. I slept with the phone. I lost weight.

I kept searching for a cure. During the next couple of months I took many bus rides to doctors, specialists, and a psychologist. Ever-changing diagnoses included: inflammation of the heart, infection of the membrane surrounding the heart, panic disorder, arrhythmia, and even cancer. Despite the highly trained medical professionals who tried to help, I had no definitive answer.

With my visa about to expire, and in worsening health, I returned to the U.S. I was so weak I had to stop and sit on the floor of the terminal several times to make it to the plane. I made it home and was hospitalized. This time, after several days in the hospital, the diagnosis was Barlow's syndrome. It meant one of my heart valves was not working properly, leading to the attacks.

The doctors prescribed medications to control my heart rate, as well as my anxiety. Healing was considered complete when my heart rate was in the normal range. Sure, the medications worked to slow down my heart, to regulate it, but they also produced side effects. These ranged from chronic tiredness to nightmares about death.

I was not living a good quality of life, even with the prescription drugs and my symptoms under control. I kept returning to what I had been pondering back in Australia. That is, I wondered if, somehow, my entire being had produced my illness. What if I had a role in being sick that went beyond medical diagnosis and treatment of symptoms? If so, then I knew I must understand how healing occurs from another vantage point.

I turned to the world of alternative medicine for an answer. Here I found a number of healing systems connected with one universal philosophy. Alternative medicine is grounded in the philosophy of *vitalism*.

Believers in vitalism believe in a vital force that permeates all life. Some call it *chi*, others *prana*, still others energy. The presence of the vital force is what separates the living from the nonliving. Alternative systems of healing work to support the vital force.

Science has a problem with vitalism. Science has never been able to measure the vital force or even a vital energy. For example, some healers say they are sending healing energy to the body, but this energy is not in any form known to science. Scientists have yet to measure a vital force, and yet, many of these healing systems still work. I, too, had a problem understanding something I could not see or measure. I thought there must be something deeper, something hiding underneath the idea of a vital force. I hoped to find some underlying process that could be explained by science that would account for the vital force.

I turned to science for an answer. Science's view of life is founded on a different philosophy than vitalism. At the core of science and medicine is mechanistic materialism. In this view life emerged from matter. There is no hidden vital force, no living energy. Life is seen as a self-sustaining process that produces complex structures. There are other processes in the universe that are capable of creating complex structures. Crystals, whirlpools, and tornadoes are examples. So what is so different about life? The vitalists would say there is no vital force in these lifeless structures.

But science, perhaps unknowingly, *does* have an answer to the mystery of the vital force. The answer lies buried deep in the process of life. It was not discovered until the middle of the twentieth century. It came from a discipline that is part science, part mathematics. This discipline is known as information theory.

Science's answer comes from the concept of information. Not information you or I may think of when we read a textbook or instruction manual, but a kind of pure information that exists all around us. It may be that behind all of the matter and energy in the universe is a ubiquitous field of information. Physicists have found such a field and call it the zero-point field (ZPF). The ZPF consists of a sea of subatomic particles popping into and out of existence. The

ZPF also produces waves that carry information faster than the speed of light. It is from this field of information that life emerged and continues to evolve to higher levels of complexity.

Life is different from nonliving systems because of its ability to capture and integrate this information from the environment. It does so with ingenious mechanisms built into all living things. For example, your body requires a constant supply of energy in order to survive. Much of this energy is in the form of an energy-carrying molecule called adenosine triphosphate (ATP). The cells of your body extract the energy from the food you eat and store it in ATP. This molecule has two primary states; one stores energy and the other releases energy. The two states of ATP contain different amounts of information. ATP contains more information in the energy-storing state. The information can then be transferred to your body. Your body uses the information to grow, and as you grow your body becomes more complex.

Life needs a constant supply of information in order to exist. If there is a lack of information or problems with information-capturing mechanisms then the organism dies.

After many years of study, two degrees, and a career as a chiropractor I finally came to the following understanding:

The essence of the vital force is information.

And

At the core of all healing systems is the transfer of information.

Information is the link between mechanistic materialism and vitalism. It is the connection between mainstream and alternative systems of healing. Healing and living are but manifestations of the same process. Illness and dying are too. All healing systems can be understood in terms of information.

My healing process was slow. It was *non-linear*; in other words my healing seemed to suddenly progress from one level to the next, in contrast to a slow, steady progress.

I received healing information from a variety of sources. These sources included medications, nutrients, herbals, a variety of mind-body healing techniques, and even my faith. Each input, although from a totally different source, was somehow able to transfer healing information to me. I integrated this information, allowing me to evolve to higher levels of functioning.

I used molecular information in the form of medications. One medication, a beta-blocker, slowed my heart rate so that it would not be so irregular. At first, I thought this would contradict the concept of supporting my physical body with healing information, since medication tends to suppress symptoms. However, my body needed a break from the constant symptoms. The medication gave me that much-needed break so that other sources of healing information could be more effective.

I supplemented the medication with other molecular sources of information, including nutrients. One nutrient I felt really helped was coenzyme Q10. This nutrient helps cells, especially heart cells, to produce energy. It has been used in the treatment of congestive heart failure with good success and is very popular in Japan. In my case it worked to support the function of my heart, allowing it to heal.

I also used information in the form of mechanical energy. I found chiropractic adjustments very helpful in allowing my body to function better. Chiropractic is based on the principle that a good functioning skeletal and muscular system will allow better information flow in the nerves and less overall stress on the body. There is much information transferred by the hands of a skilled practitioner.

I used my mind as an information source by practicing a number of mind-body healing techniques such as creative visualization and imagery. The mind can be a very powerful source of healing information as it connects to virtually every part of your body via the neuro-endocrine system. I also made a connection to higher levels of information through healing intention. This allowed for the instantaneous transfer of information from consciousness.

Eventually I progressed to a state of healing wherein my symptoms diminished, then disappeared completely. I evolved to a level of functioning in which I no longer had the problem. The process took about ten years. I noticed that my symptoms were not the only problems missing. My entire life was better, more improved, more satisfying.

Many of the old behavior patterns that led to my illness were gone. My thinking had become clearer and less dysfunctional. There was a profound change at the core of my being. This change on such a deep level resulted from a kind of learning that came with the infusion of information.

My healing was confirmed a few years after graduating from professional college when a number of medical tests revealed that everything was normal. My healing did not mark the end of my journey, but the beginning of a new phase. I wanted to learn more about the process of information transfer.

During this new phase of my journey I had the opportunity to speak with health-care practitioners of many disciplines. I could sense the excitement in their voices when they told me of their successes with patients. What struck me was that they *all had successes*. Once I understood healing in terms of information, I began to see that all these healing systems were in essence the same. All involved the transfer of information. I also gained a greater understanding of my own healing. I had integrated this information from all of these sources and evolved to a higher level of functioning, *without the disease*.

I set out to develop a system of healing based on the transfer of information. So far it has taken me six years to do so. I am constantly working on the system and incorporating it in my practice of chiropractic. This book is the result and presents a system of healing that can be used by anyone. It integrates ideas from physics, molecular biology, medicine, psychoneuroimmunology, alternative healing, and information theory. It contains many of the techniques I have personally used in my own healing and with patients. It presents a unified theory of healing that explains mainstream and alternative systems of healing in terms of one underlying process. All healing systems encompass the flow of information, regardless of whether the practitioner is an MD from Yale or a shaman from Tibet.

I call this new system of healing *informational healing*. Informational healing consists of seven principles that I refer to as *keys*. Healing information is all around us but in order to use it effectively we need to understand and use the keys. The keys allow us to tap into this unlimited supply of healing information. The keys are introduced in chapter three. Chapters one and two provide important background information needed to understand the keys.

An important concept is that healing information flows from a source to a receiver through a channel. Chapter four tells you how to resonate with sources of healing information. Chapters five through ten describe each healing channel in detail and include exercises to help you to make the best use of each channel.

One of the main goals of this book is to provide a system of healing that anyone can use. Chapter eleven pulls the entire system together by presenting a step-by-step approach. There is an easy-to-follow flowchart and set of worksheets to help you along. Finally, chapter thirteen explores the future direction of informational healing.

This book is written for anyone needing to heal. You can take the concepts presented here and apply them immediately. You will also find this book useful in understanding, evaluating, and designing healing programs that integrate both mainstream and alternative systems of healing. We are entering a new realm of understanding our universe in terms of information and we need to apply this new revelation to healing. When this happens we will move toward a more complete system of healing, one in which practitioners of all systems can communicate and work toward the common goal of developing a unified system of healing.

CHAPTER I

DAY OF THE CADAVERS

It was a hot and humid Texas day. There we were, the new class of first-trimester chiropractic students nervously waiting outside the brick concrete building that housed the gross anatomy lab. We tried not to let the already sweltering conditions disturb our fragile states of composure. Today was the day we were to begin our dissection class. We were eager, excited, and a little frightened of what this experience would bring. I looked over my classmates. It was this class that would test our mettle. It was this class that would determine whether we had what it took to move forward in our pursuit of new careers. I wondered who of us would not make it through the day, much less the entire two-semester course.

Dr. Sami appeared on the other side of the glass doors. He quickly unlocked them and ushered us in. "Welcome gentlemen ... *and* ladies," he said with a strong Indian accent. We made a makeshift, single-file line and proceeded past the thick glass doors. I had walked by the lab a few days ago and peered in, only to see a tile wall holding the school insignia. The real mysteries were around the corner and out of sight. I had wondered what it was like in there. How many bodies were there? Were they exposed? Would it shock me to see them? How bad did it smell in there? These and many more questions raced through my mind.

As we walked in and turned the corner I felt that each step took me closer to the answers to my questions. There beyond the tile wall was a large, open room. A narrow, rectangular bank of windows adorned the uppermost section of the walls. There were rows of the familiar fluorescent lights. The concrete floor looked very clean. The only smell in the air was a mild chemical smell, nothing like what I had expected. Positioned around the room were a dozen stainless-steel tanks. Each tank had some valves and levers attached to it. Each tank was on wheels. "So far so good," I thought to myself. No bodies yet and the smell wasn't so bad.

"Everyone count off by five," Dr. Sami said. The students responded accordingly. I ended up being a two. Dr. Sami pointed to the first row of tanks on the right side of the room and said, "Ones over here." The group of "ones" stood around the tank. Dr. Sami walked to the second tank and said, "Twos over here." I and the other "twos" gathered around the tank. The remaining students were assigned to their respective tanks.

During this ritual Dr. Sami's lab assistants had appeared. One disappeared into a room behind the teacher's desk. The other stood next to Dr. Sami. "This is Bill. He's one of the lab techs here in the gross lab, Pete is back in the freezer. Now you go to get your body. One's first…" he said with a more authoritative voice. Bill stepped in and directed the operation from here on out. The "ones" were assigned a male, we "twos" a female, and so on. The first tank disappeared into the "freezer" room with Pete. A few minutes later it was our turn. We pushed the tank toward the room and as we neared the entrance the "ones" emerged with a large body bag in their tank. I caught a glimpse of as they passed. We entered the freezer. It was markedly colder in there, but not cold enough for anything to actually freeze. Along one wall was a large structure that looked like a makeshift shelving unit. It reminded me of those crime stories on television in which someone goes to the morgue to identify a body. The body is usually inside a storage unit with a door. The coroner opens the door and slides out the body.

This structure was similar but there were no doors, just square cubicle-like shelves. Some were empty and others held body bags. We spotted Pete, who had climbed halfway up the shelves. "Last group got a male, you get a female," he said as he jockeyed about the shelves. He stopped at one and after checking its contents said, "Here we go. I need a little help here." We looked at each other and my classmate and I moved closer. Pete grabbed the bag and began to pull it out of the cubicle. We tentatively grabbed the bag and helped Pete pull the remainder of the body out. The bag was very heavy and hard to maneuver. There was fluid sloshing around inside. The other twos joined us in placing the bag and its contents into our tank. We proceeded back to our station in the lab.

Pete was now out of the freezer and helping out with the groups. He came over to our group and told us to remove our body from the bag. One of us took a scalpel and cut the thick, blue plastic bag away. There she was, our cadaver. "We will be spending a lot of time together," I thought to myself.

I took a good look at the body. Her arms and legs were tied with heavy twine. "That's how they move them … with a hoist," said Pete. I noticed she looked very old and frail, maybe close to eighty years old. There were no surgical scars except for the severed carotid and femoral arteries where they infused the embalming fluid. The chemical smell became even stronger and it caused our faces to itch.

I noticed her face. She had the look of someone who was asleep. I assumed her facial expression was what she had at the time of her death. Not only was her body preserved but also her experience of death was recorded by her features. I looked around the room at the other cadavers. Some had a similar sleeping expression but others had an expression of pain. There was one in particular, a male, who had a grimace as if his last few moments were spent in excruciating pain. Others had a more peaceful look.

Many thoughts raced through my head. Here I was, face-to-face with death. Here I was, alive, standing over this dead person. I had only been exposed to death once before in my life. An elderly lady had collapsed at a skating rink and died shortly after. I was dating a nurse who had administered CPR at the time during the moments before the ambulance came. The feeling I had at that time in my young life was to escape the scene. I wanted nothing to do with death.

Now, here I was, face-to-face with death again, but this time there was no escape. Not only did I have to get through today's lab, but there were two more five-hour sessions this week and every week thereafter for the better part of a year. No, there was no escaping this scene. Here I was, not only exposed to death, but having to dissect it, to pick it apart piece by piece, so that I could learn about life. I felt a sense of gratitude to our cadaver lady for donating her body.

As the other groups of students opened their bags I noticed a decrease in the noise level in the lab. My fellow classmates were talking in a lowered voice as if at a funeral. An automatic response of respect for the deceased, I thought. One of the other students in my group suggested we name her. He suggested "Evelyn." "She looks like an Evelyn," he said. We agreed on his choice.

This class marked the beginning of my fascinating journey into the complexity of the human body. After the initial few exposures to the cadaver I soon became used to the sights, sounds, and smells of the cadaver lab. I was there for every open lab period as well. My focus during that first year of study was to learn as much about the body as possible. There were days of intense frustration and tedium as each layer of tissue was carefully separated. These were countered with days of wondrous exploration and discovery. I learned something with each session; each slice of the scalpel, each scissoring of tissue gave me knowledge I would not have gained through textbooks or lectures. To work on a real body is a real privilege. Not everyone has an experience such as this.

I often thought about the difference between the living and the non-living. I had seen dead things before, but I never gave it much thought. Now I was struck with the idea that the body I worked on was nothing but a shell. It was as if time stood still for this person. Here were all of the body systems frozen in time there for me to examine—none of which would ever work again. This body was slowly decaying. The strong chemicals it contained worked to keep the process of decay at bay.

I later learned the rather morbid concept that all things in this universe eventually decay. It is a fundamental law given the name of *entropy*. Every tissue, molecule, and atom is subject to this law. Everything will eventually become disorganized to the point of nonexistence, in a hopeless sequence of events from which there is no escape. There is *no* escape from entropy. I found it difficult to accept this rather nihilistic view of our existence. I began my study of living systems from the point of view of entropy and found something quite wondrous and hopeful. I found that living beings actually thwart the immutable law of entropy.

I discovered that even though the universe continues to evolve to a state of greater *disorganization*, living beings evolve to states of greater *organization*. During their lifetimes, living beings fly in the face of entropy. Life on Earth, as a whole, also evolves to higher states of organization. From infinitesimal chemical systems to viruses and bacteria, to plants, insects, animals, and humans, life on Earth continues a process of increasing organization.

But how can this be? How can life, an ordered system, emerge and exist in a system of increasing disorder? These questions puzzled scientists and philosophers for generations. In the philosophical camp called vitalism, vitalists believed in a vital force, a life force that permeated all living beings. The vital force was what kept things alive, but no one was ever able to measure this mysterious force.

After hundreds of years of study, science finally found an answer to the emergence of order in living beings. Science found that life was able to do something unique regarding entropy. Life has the ability to capture something special from the environment. That special *something* allows life to counter entropy. It is what keeps living beings alive and allows life to evolve to higher states of complexity. That something is *information.*

Not the information you may think of in reading a newspaper or working out a math problem, but a kind of knowledge that permeates the universe. Everything contains different amounts of information. The molecules in our food, the energy from the sun, even the air we breathe contains information.

The more complex something is, the more information it contains. A simple molecule of water does not contain as much information with its two atoms of hydrogen and one atom of oxygen as, say, a protein with its hundred amino acid molecules. The protein also contains hydrogen and oxygen atoms, but their arrangement is different, they have a different *relationship.* Information has to do with *relationships.* It has to do with how things are put together. Information is inherent in the structure of things.

Information is very real. Matter, energy, and information are all connected. Einstein first made the connection between energy and matter with his famous equation: $E = mc^2$. E represents the energy, m is the mass of a substance, and c^2 is the speed of light (300,000 kilometers per second). Einstein discovered that matter and energy are equivalent and that very large amounts of energy can be extracted from very small amounts of matter.

The connection between energy and information wasn't found until the 1960s. The discovery was made in computer science by the physicist Rolf Landauer and had to do with the way a computer stores information. A computer stores information in its memory. This memory may be a silicon chip or a magnetic tape. It turns out that information can be stored in a computer's memory without using or releasing energy into the universe. We can even manipulate information without a net increase or decrease in energy. But there is one operation that releases energy into the universe and it is impossible to perform any kind of meaningful information processing without it. Landauer found that you cannot *erase* information without releasing energy into the universe (increasing its entropy).

The importance of Landauer's discovery is the link between information and energy. Energy and information are as closely linked as matter and energy. When combined with Einstein's formula we see that information, energy, and matter are all linked together. Just as a given quantity of matter holds a certain amount of energy, that energy also contains a certain amount of information. Information is not a theoretical concept but a physical thing.

Erwin Schrödinger, a famous physicist who was fascinated with life, put forth a valuable insight regarding life and information. Schrödinger was one of the pioneers of a branch of physics called quantum mechanics. Quantum mechanics was a revolutionary discovery in that it changed the way we view matter, energy, and even reality. Schrödinger was a key player in developing this revolutionary science. Schrödinger's fascination with life and living systems inspired a series of lectures that became an important book titled *What is Life?* In this book he said that life is characterized by the "ability to create order from disorder by exploiting external energy sources (negative entropy)."[1]

Schrödinger's statement gets us closer to the essence of the underlying process of life. Somehow, life emerged in a universe of ever-increasing disorder. Biological molecules had the uncanny ability to assemble themselves in such a way as to create highly ordered systems. Living systems were capable of evolving by means of capturing and integrating what Schrödinger called negative entropy. The negative entropy he refers to is *information*. All matter and energy are somehow put together as if from a set of relationships. Life somehow captures the essence of these relationships. The information exists within our being; it is in the atoms and molecules of our bodies. It is even in our consciousness.

As we continued our dissection of Evelyn we studied all of the major body systems. At one time these systems must have been teeming with the flow of information. Evelyn's respiratory system took in oxygen and released carbon dioxide. These molecules were distributed throughout her body by the heart and blood vessels. When she exercised, her nervous system sensed the need for more oxygen and caused her to breathe heavier and faster. Her heart pumped with greater speed and force. Her cells produced more energy. All of her body systems were dependent on one another. All of her systems communicated by transferring information.

Information is exchanged among all body systems and all levels of organization. It flows from cell to cell and system to system in a concert of activity we know as life. Information is needed to sustain life, to keep the omnipresent second law of thermodynamics at bay. It is needed to reduce the entropy of the human body and of all life.

To live is to gather and integrate information.

Throughout our lives we continue to gather and integrate the information around us. It may be in the form of the structure of the molecules of the food we eat or the energy of the sun. It may even be more ethereal, in the form of the connections of cells in our brains that produce our behaviors. The information we gather keeps us in a state that is out of balance. In science we say this is a nonequilibrium state. It is only at death that we reach equilibrium. All information gathering ceases and we join the rest of the nonliving in a process of decay.

When I think about my time with Evelyn I realize that her body was at equilibrium while I existed in a state of nonequilibrium. As we continued our dissection we discovered that she had cancer. We found it in the lymph nodes under her arms; we found it in her lungs and liver. It had even manifested as dark spots in her bones. We had no training in pathology or diseases at the time of our dissection class, but we intuitively knew it was cancer. We could tell by the different look of the cancerous tissue. Organ tissue normally looks symmetrical with nice borders. The cancerous tissue was discolored and asymmetrical with hard-to-define borders. The cancerous tissue was greatly disorganized.

Cancerous cells begin to produce faulty instructions and send them to other cells. In some cases, the DNA is unable to correct these errors resulting in an interruption of the normal flow of information needed to sustain the cells. Instead of maintaining organization, cancerous cells cause disorganization and mutate wildly.

The same thing occurs with the common cold. Viruses attack and enter our cells, taking them over and causing them to manufacture more virus. The virus causes disorganization in the body. We experience this as a cold.

Our immune systems are instrumental in allowing us to get over or heal from colds. Immune cells recognize the virus as a threat and attack it. Immune cells also form an information network to communicate with each other. The entire immune response is a concert of information flow. Information is infused into the body, and the body again moves toward greater complexity. The body heals.

Evelyn had succumbed to a great degree of disorganization or entropy in her body. The concerted flow of information was severely disrupted. Eventually the entropy had taken over and she had passed on. In contrast, we students had bodies that kept entropy at bay. Somehow our bodies could capture enough information to slow the process of entropy.

Evelyn was born with a well-functioning body, which was evident by her advanced age. She must have had a good life up until near the end. Her body must have been able to collect and integrate information in order to maintain her health, at least until the cancer.

Our bodies always work to sustain us and decrease entropy by constantly infusing information. Illness occurs when the body moves toward death (increased entropy). We can apply this concept to health and healing. We can think of healing as the flow of information to the systems of the body in order to reduce entropy. Illness, on the other hand can be defined as a movement of the body toward a state of disorganization.

I still have the privilege of working on cadavers in the capacity of a teacher of anatomy and physiology to my allied health students. I have learned something from each cadaver and am grateful for the experience. Occasionally a student will ask about my first dissection class and I will tell the story of Evelyn. In a way she has given me much; in a way she lives on and continues to do so through my teachings and what my students pass on to others.

This idea of <u>healing as exchanges of information</u> leaves many unanswered questions. Where does the information come from? How can it be used to heal? Can anybody use it? Is it difficult to use? The remainder of this book is devoted to providing answers to these questions and more.

CHAPTER 2

INFORMATION STRUCTURES AND CHANNELS

Years ago I lived near the ocean. I often found it relaxing to go to the beach to just sit and watch the waves and listen to the surf. Waves always fascinated me; particularly how each wave was unique. I would think how amazing it was that this giant structure of the ocean was capable of producing an infinite variety of waves. Not only were waves possible, but an infinite variety of smaller phenomena such as whirlpools and currents were also possible.

We can think of the ocean as a vast informational structure. The ocean is not only vast, but also very complex. Contained within it are a myriad of other, less complex structures such as currents, whirlpools, and waves. In order for these smaller structures to exist, there must be some sort of communication from the larger ocean structure. For example, a whirlpool forms at the end of a traveling wave for a few brief moments. It appears that the force of the wave supports the whirlpool. This is true, but if we look deeper—if we look to see what is happening behind the force—we see that there is something else. What supports the whirlpool is information.

<u>Force is, in essence, information</u>. There is communication of information from the ocean to the smaller waves and whirlpools. The flow of information from the ocean supports the waves and whirlpools. Eventually the flow ceases as these smaller structures are not stable enough to support themselves. Their brief lives mark periods of organization within a system of flowing water that seems disorganized. For a short time they exist as complex structures, only to break apart, consumed once again by the ocean.

Our universe is much like an ocean. Information flows between structures of varying complexity. We, too, are informational structures. Information flows to us to support our existence and our health. Like the whirlpool, we need a continuous supply of information from other sources in order to keep us alive.

There are many ways to organize structures according to information. Our concern, however, is with living and healing, so I have organized the structures with this in mind. They are organized according to gross levels of complexity. All of the levels have an effect on our lives. All are potential sources of healing information.

I will call this organization of structures the information hierarchy. There are six broad categories of information, as shown in figure 2.1.

The zero-point field is at the top of the hierarchy and represents the most complex structure. This field permeates our universe and everything in it. It connects everything in a web of reality and transmits information faster than the speed of light. It also may contain a record of all events in the universe.

Physicists have discovered that space is not continuous, as was once thought. At the most minute levels, space is not smooth but alive with activity. Particles continuously pop into existence, then combine and annihilate each other. The field carries the name zero-point because, over time, the activity statistically cancels out. However, at any one instant of time, space is alive with energy.

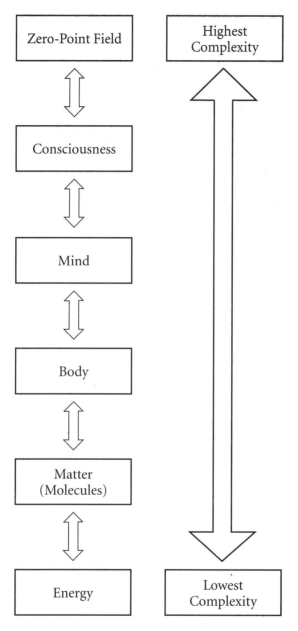

Figure 2.1 The information hierarchy. Levels of information are presented according to their corresponding complexity. Tiny energy particles constitute the lowest level while the zero-point field represents the highest level.

Physicists have been searching for a field of this nature for quite some time. Experiments conducted in the early part of the twentieth century revealed an energy source existing at a temperature of near absolute zero (another reason for the name zero-point). The experiments consisted of first creating a vacuum in an area insulated from electromagnetic radiation. The experiments were then cooled to near absolute zero where there is no movement of molecules, and the search for energy began. What was remarkable was that instead of finding no energy the experimenters found huge amounts of energy—energy that seemed to come out of nothing!

Besides containing vast amounts of energy, the zero-point field also carries information. It does so by virtue of pressure waves, called quantum vacuum waves. This means that the entire universe is connected by an immense information network. This network produces matter and energy out of seemingly empty space. A number of scientists support this idea, including Nobel prize nominee Ervin László. In his book, *Science and the Akashic Field*, he discusses the properties of these waves:

> *The vacuum could indeed have such a property. It could be not just a superdense sea of energy, but also a sea of information.*[1]

The network is capable of communicating information faster than the speed of light, which is virtually impossible in physics. A few physicists have investigated this phenomenon. According to physicist Gennady Shipov, these vacuum waves carry information at $10^9 c$, or one billion times greater than the speed of light.[2]

All subsequent lower-level informational structures are imbedded in the zero-point field. Like the whirlpools and waves in the ocean, smaller structures must have some sort of communication of information from the zero-point field. Information must travel from one point to another. I will call this connection a *channel*. The source produces the information and the channel carries it. In the ocean example the channel consists of water molecules transferring force from one to another. The information is contained in the physical characteristics of the force such as mass and velocity. The zero-point field transfers information across a channel, but the medium is much different. The medium consists of the quantum vacuum waves.

Just below the zero-point field is the next level in the hierarchy: consciousness. Quantum physics tells us that consciousness has a causative effect on matter. In quantum physics objects exist first as probabilities, until observed by consciousness. For example, light exists as both waves and particles until observed. Once consciousness observes the light, it becomes either a wave or particle. The probability no longer exists. We call this the collapse of the probability wave. The light now has a context, a more concrete form.

Consciousness somehow chooses to see a wave or a particle. By doing so it gives the situation meaning; it puts it into context; it makes a decision. The decision is a powerful means for transferring information. Decisions can be thought of as information in action.

A number of scientists have proposed theories regarding the transfer of information from structure such as the zero-point field or consciousness to structures that exist in physical form. One of these scientists is biologist Rupert Sheldrake who has developed an idea he calls the hypothesis of formative causation. He says that the physical form of living things emerges from what he calls a morphogenetic field. The morphogenetic field contains the information needed to direct the manifestation and development of living things. The field tells the living system what form to take. The field is also capable of carrying information and transferring it to future generations.

He states:

> I suggest that morphogenetic fields work by imposing patterns on otherwise random or indeterminate patterns of activity.[3]

Sheldrake's morphogenetic field is an information field from which life emerges. Psychologist Carl Jung also spoke of a similar field he called the collective unconscious. Jung indicated that we are all connected via the collective unconscious. According to Jung, the collective unconscious stores memories of all human events. Jung thought that memories were not stored in our physical brains, but in some field-like entity that is accessible by all humans.

Physicist Amit Goswami speaks of consciousness as an intermediary between the morphogenetic field and physical form. He believes the physical body is a representation of the morphogenetic field. He states:

… the morphogenetic fields that the physical body organs represent. Once the representations are made, the organs run the programs that carry out the biological functions. The representation maker, the programmer, is consciousness.[4]

Sheldrake's morphogenetic field is an information field that exists within the zero-point field. It imposes patterns through the communication of information into biological systems. Goswami's view adds consciousness to the picture as an intermediary between the morphogenetic field and physical form. I will place the morphogenetic field at the same level of consciousness in the hierarchy. There are two reasons for doing this. First, little is known about the structure of information in consciousness, and the morphogenetic field or about quantum vacuum waves. We know there is a connection, but we don't know much about the details. Second, we are concerned with the transfer of healing information. As far as we know, information at this level is transferred nonlocally, a phenomenon we will explore further in chapter five. Information from the morphogenetic field and consciousness is transferred the same way.

The next lower step in the hierarchy is the mind. The mind is the link between our physical bodies and the outer world. Our minds continually take in information from our surroundings and experiences and put it into contextual form. The mind then controls the body through the neuroendocrine system.

The mind is an informational source just like all of the levels in the hierarchy. The receiver of the mind's information is the body. The channel is the neuroendocrine system, a complex network of nerve cells and hormones. The system is intimately connected to every part of our physical bodies.

Our bodies represent the physical manifestation of our existence. I have placed the body just below the mind in the hierarchy. Our bodies are our vessels for our earthly journeys through life. In healing we ultimately want to heal our bodies. The body is the midpoint in the hierarchy. It is the receiver of information from the sources above and below in the hierarchy.

The lowest levels in the hierarchy are matter and energy. These are the simplest informational structures we know. Matter consists of fundamental particles such as protons, neutrons, and electrons, which themselves consist of smaller particles called *quarks*. Energy consists of forces that also consist of particles. The particles are exchanged between matter particles. For example one of the four fundamental forces, the electromagnetic force, is carried by photons.

Energy and matter particles can be thought of as tiny individual packets of information. These particles differ in information content from the collective nature of the particles in the zero-point field. In the zero-point field, the particles are like the entire ocean in our example above, whereas matter and energy particles are like the individual water molecules in the ocean.

During our lives, information flows from all of the structures in the hierarchy to our bodies. Downward causation occurs when information flows from structures located at higher levels in the hierarchy to the body. The information has a causative effect on the body. For example, a problem with the mind such as depression or negative self-image can have a negative effect on the body.

Likewise, the lower structures in the hierarchy can affect the body. Information flowing from molecules and energy to the body can have a positive or negative effect. This is called upward causation. Figure 2.2 illustrates the concept of upward and downward causation on the body.

Many alternative systems of healing affect the higher levels in the hierarchy such as consciousness and the mind. Thus, alternative systems work by virtue of downward causation. For example, Reiki may work by transferring information to consciousness that produces a downward causation to heal the physical body. Other systems of healing such as traditional Chinese medicine and Ayurveda also work on the higher levels to produce changes in the lower levels of physical

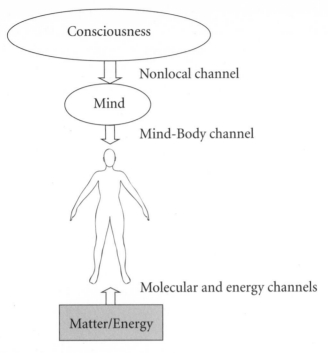

Figure 2.2 The downward causation of consciousness and mind and the upward causation of matter and energy on the body.

existence. Generally, systems of healing based on vitalism work this way.

Mainstream medicine (allopathy) is mostly concerned with upward causation. Allopathy primarily uses the lower levels of the hierarchy, molecules and energy, to affect the body. Evoking a change on these lower levels causes changes in the upper levels. Medications work by upward causation. Molecules in medications can evoke changes in cells and tissues that translate to the higher level of the body.

For example the drug Paxil (paroxetine) is used to treat depression. Paxil works by blocking the degradation of the neurotransmitter serotonin. Serotonin has been linked to some types of depressions— serotonin levels are low in some depressed individuals. Blocking the degradation of serotonin causes a rise in serotonin levels that decreases the symptoms of depression. Depression has a global effect on the body. It not only causes negative moods but can also cause physical symptoms such as lethargy and muscle pain that can render an individual disabled. The molecular information provided by Paxil/ paroxetine then has a global effect on the body. The small amount of information contained in the drug has the potential to change the much larger informational structure of the body.

Most of the textbooks I use for teaching my classes in anatomy and physiology describe life in terms of upward causation. There are increasing levels of complexity built from lower levels, with the lower levels affecting the higher. Atoms combine to form molecules that combine to form cells, tissues, organs, and systems.

However, visionaries like Sheldrake and Goswami stress the importance of downward causation and its effects on life. We are more than an assemblage of atoms and molecules. Our existence extends to the upper reaches of the hierarchy and information from these higher sources has an effect on our existence. When we heal we must address all levels of our existence.

The hierarchy allows us to unify all systems of healing and to explain phenomena that occur in alternative systems of healing. We have the allopathic approach with its emphasis on the upward causation of molecules (medicines) causing healing changes in the body. We also have the alternative methods with their emphasis on the downward causation of consciousness and mind healing the body.

The Four Informational Healing Channels

The system of informational healing consists of four channels, each of which represents a connection to the different levels of the information hierarchy. Figure 2.3 illustrates the four healing channels.

The mind and consciousness communicate with the zero-point field. The transfer of information between them occurs through what I will call the nonlocal channel. No one knows just how this information transfer occurs. We do know that it does occur and this effect has been substantiated by considerable research (see chapter five).

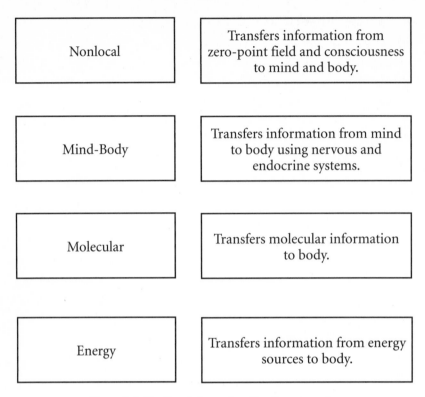

Figure 2.3 The four informational healing channels.

The mind is also an information source that transfers information to the body through what I will call the mind-body channel. This channel is more concrete than the nonlocal channel as it is an actual physical system in the body. The mind-body channel is the neuroendocrine system. I will describe the mind-body channel in chapter seven.

The molecular channel is the medium through which molecular information flows. Molecular information is contained in medications, nutrients, herbals, and biologicals. In most cases the molecular channel is the circulatory system that carries this information to target tissues such as organs or glands.

This energy channel carries information in the form of force particles. The channel is the medium through which the force particles travel. This could be air in the case of sound waves, space in the case of light, and body tissue in the case of mechanical pressure.

The informational healing system involves the use of all four channels in order to infuse the body with healing information. We exist as energy, molecules, mind, and consciousness, so we must heal on each of these levels. We will do this by using sources of information for each level with the goal of providing as much healing information as possible to our bodies.

CHAPTER 3

UNLOCKING THE CODE

We need a constant supply of information in order to survive and heal. Information is everywhere; we only need to learn how to access it in order to heal. The information is there to help us but it is not directly accessible. It is encoded, locked up in a secret code that requires a special set of keys. The keys are the principles of informational healing presented here.

Before presenting the keys, we need to better understand the role of information flow in healing by looking at a few examples. In these examples the word *disorganization* has the same meaning as *entropy*.

First, let's look at the vascular system. Blood flows though the body, picking up oxygen from the lungs and transporting it to the cells and tissues. There are many systems of the body working together to maintain the blood pressure to move blood to where it is needed. The vascular system works with the nervous, endocrine, and urinary systems to keep the pressure constant. All can be thought of as an organized system; a system with a high degree of complexity.

Now let's say there is an injury, a serious laceration. There is a good amount of bleeding. Instead of blood flowing to the cells and tissues, it flows out of the body. The system now suffers from disorganization.

The body responds to the disorganization by attempting to move in the direction of organization. The nervous system causes blood vessels to constrict; the kidneys shut down and release hormones to conserve blood. Even the blood has systems built into it to counteract the bleeding. The blood forms a clot to plug the hole in the vessel. All of these systems work to reorganize the vascular system. If they are successful the body heals, if not the body moves toward greater disorganization and eventually death.

This movement toward organization is commonly called *homeostasis.* Homeostasis is the body's ability to maintain a level of something such as calcium or glucose in the blood by incorporating the use of feedback systems. The system senses a change in the level and responds by activating a mechanism to bring it back to where it should be. Homeostasis is what keeps us alive. It is what keeps all of the systems in our bodies working together in harmony. Our hearts beat at just the right rate in order to provide just the right amount of blood, carrying just the right amount of oxygen to the tissues. Our brains require a constant supply of glucose, which is carefully provided by the hormones of the endocrine system. Too much or too little glucose would result in a coma. All of the internal systems of the body are kept in a delicate balance.

Homeostasis does not operate without a constant influx of information. As the level of a substance changes, information must be sent to a regulating system so that it can react. The regulating system must also react to the change in some way that involves information.

In our bleeding example there is a change in the body, a movement toward entropy. Homeostatic mechanisms must react by infusing information into the system to move it back so the system can again become organized. For example the nervous system senses the falling blood pressure. It reacts by sending information to the blood vessels

Key 1: Use Healing Intention First.

Key 2: Healing information flows from a source to a receiver through a channel.

Key 3: Use all four informational healing channels.

Key 4: The information source and receiver must resonate.

Key 5: Your consciousness automatically seeks healing information.

Key 6: A hierarchy of information sources.

Key 7: Fine-tune information flow with feedback.

Figure 3.1 The seven informational healing keys.

to constrict in an attempt to maintain the pressure. The kidneys also sense the falling pressure and release hormones that are analogous to tiny packets of information. They tell the kidneys to shut down and hold on to the volume of blood. All of the systems work to maintain the pressure by infusing information into the broken system.

Another example is the disorganized nature of cancer cells. Normal cells exhibit a high degree of organization. When they divide, they produce exact copies and form very organized systems that work in concert to perform various functions. Cancer cells exhibit a high degree of disorganization. When they divide they produce mutations that drastically alter the normal functions. They are also capable of moving throughout the body, subsequently spreading disorganization everywhere.

The body works to overcome increasing entropy the best it can. The body's systems work to reorganize the damaged cells by infusing information. Sometimes it is successful at doing so and sometimes it is not.

There are many more examples of homeostasis and the infusion of information into body systems to bring them back into a more organized state. The main point is that it takes information to maintain homeostasis and subsequently to heal.

There are seven keys to unlocking the healing code. Figure 3.1 illustrates all seven keys. Together they constitute a powerful system of healing and will help you to use a limitless supply of healing information. These keys can also be applied to virtually any type of healing and integrate all healing systems. It is important to work to generally understand each key before moving on to the remainder of the book. Feel free to revisit this section as necessary to review the keys.

Key #1: Use Healing Intention First

This is probably the most important concept in using informational healing, and the simplest. You need not visit any practitioner, take any medication, vitamin, herb, or expose yourself to any modality. You simply need to have the intention to heal. This sounds simple enough, but there are cases when this can be very difficult.

When we are ill, we need to activate all the healing channels and focus the information on our problem. Healing intention helps us to do so. Besides providing a purpose to our actions, healing intention opens up the nonlocal information channel to send healing information to us instantaneously. We will discuss the use of the nonlocal channel in chapters five and six.

Intention provides focus to healing. Any interference with intention also interferes with healing. Sometimes interference manifests as a deep-down wish to remain ill. I have seen this many times in practice with patients. Sometimes people define themselves in terms of their illnesses. The attention they receive somehow fills a need. Perhaps they are looking for a way to get out of a bad personal situation or job, and illness gives them a reason to do so. I have found that these people tend to resist treatments. In some cases this tendency becomes so extreme it feels like a contest between the patient and myself. Whatever I suggest to help them is met with reasons for why it will not work. These people need to reflect on their illness so they may get at some deeper issues that may be supporting the illness. Chapter six provides some exercises for doing this.

Masking an illness can interfere with intention. For example, flu sufferers may continue to abuse their bodies with poor diets, overwork, and stress. They may think that a symptom-suppressing medication is enough to allow them to heal.

Doubt also interferes with intention. If you truly doubt a treatment ,it may be best to avoid it. The same goes for faith in your practitioner. Intuition can go a long way in helping to make these decisions.

Practitioners too must operate from an intention to heal. Healing is not a contest to be won by the practitioner. It is important to work with patients, not to prove them wrong. This is especially important for practitioners of disparate healing systems such as medicine, homeopathy, chiropractic, acupuncture, naturopathy, and so on. I have personally experienced the full array of responses from the medical establishment in my practice of chiropractic, from being referred to as a "quack" to full respect regarding my contributions to the treatment of a patient.

It is important to support the patient's decision to see other health-care providers. I have seen alternative practitioners discount the medical system. Practitioners must work to understand that there is truth in both systems of healing. Information is the common component of all healing systems. Keep an open mind and educate yourself if necessary about the other modalities patients are using.

Key #2: Healing Information Flows From a Source to a Receiver Through a Channel

In order to infuse information into a system, there must be a source. I will present a number of sources of healing information throughout this book. The information emanating from the source travels to the receiver. The receiver is the person, tissues, or cells needing to heal. In order for the information to get to the receiver it must travel through a channel (see chapter two). The channel has a set capacity to handle a certain amount of information. If the source is too weak, information may be lost; if too strong it may exceed the channel's capacity and become distorted.

Key #3: Use All Four Informational Healing Channels

Healing information flows through four channels. These are the molecular, energy, mind-body, and nonlocal channels. The molecular channel carries information from molecule to molecule such as when using vitamins, minerals, herbs, and medicines. The energy channel carries information in the form of forces, primarily the electromagnetic force. Some examples of forces include light, electricity, magnetism, and mechanical force.

Our own minds can send healing information to our bodies through the mind-body channel. Our mind interprets the information from our senses, integrates it, and gives it meaning. Information is sent from the mind to the body through the neuroendocrine system.

Lastly, information travels through a mysterious nonlocal channel. This channel is the strangest channel of all, as information travels faster than the speed of light. You can send nonlocal information using the zero-point field.

It is best to use all four information channels if possible. Most of us typically use only one channel to provide healing information. This may not be enough, as healing occurs on all of the levels. Also, when you use more than one channel you will find you will need to rely on one information source less.

Not only can you use more than one channel, but you can use more than one information source for each channel as well. Many people rely on just one information source to heal. For example, I have seen patients who relied on one medication, one herbal supplement, or one modality such as physical therapy or massage. Once I began using more information sources and channels, I found I had to use each individual one less. In many cases patients decreased their reliance on medications or other treatments. The key is to use *all* of the channels, in contrast to using many sources for *one* channel.

Key #4: The Information Source and Receiver Must Resonate

All channels are capable of carrying a certain amount of information. All channels also contain interference or noise. The noise must be overcome in order to get the information through the channel.

The strength of the source must match the resistance of the receiver as closely as possible to overcome noise in the channel. If the source is too weak, not enough information gets through to promote healing; if too strong, it overpowers the receiver. When source and receiver match, they resonate with healing information.

Key #5: Your Consciousness Automatically Seeks Healing Information

Your consciousness is very adept at becoming aware of disturbances in the organization of your body. When you are ill, your consciousness seeks healing information. This happens automatically without any effort on your part. There is a caveat, however, and that is that you will sometimes need to get in touch with your need to seek healing information in order to allow it to flow.

Key #6: A Hierarchy of Information Sources

Information exists at different levels (see chapter two). At the highest level there is pure information. Pure information exists in the zero-point field.

Consciousness represents the next highest order of information. Consciousness connects the zero-point field with the mind, which is the next level below consciousness. The mind is the link between consciousness and the body. Matter and energy, our lowest levels of information, also communicate with the body.

There generally appears to be an inverse relationship between the hierarchy of information and the strength of its effect on the body. For example, nonlocal information from consciousness has a weaker effect on molecules than does information from other molecules. In other words you would be less successful in trying to change the information in a molecule through meditation versus medication or nutrients. Perhaps this inverse relationship results from the order of complexity of information present in the physical body. Healing occurs on a number of levels corresponding to the hierarchical order of information.

However, healing goes deeper than the physical realm. Healing occurs on other levels such as in the mind and consciousness. For example, one can heal the mind while the body is experiencing physical illness. Or, to enter the realm of consciousness, one can heal the consciousness while the mind and body are experiencing illness. This is why all the healing channels should be used.

Key #7: Fine-tune Information Flow with Feedback

Feedback occurs when the product of a process is integrated into the process and contributes to its function. Feedback allows informational systems to fine-tune their information gathering and integration processes. There must be a purpose to the process, and feedback accelerates the movement of the system toward this purpose. Our bleeding example is one of the thousands of feedback systems in the body that work together to maintain homeostasis.

Feedback is also important in healing. It can be very subtle. Feedback can be used with all four healing channels. To begin to use feedback there must be some initial measurement of the problem. This measurement is then monitored for signs of progress.

Practitioners can provide feedback through continuous monitoring of the healing response and adjustment of the treatment as needed. This is usually done every time the patient is seen.

Anyone can use feedback. One excellent way to do so is to use a healing journal. It is best to quantify results if at all possible. Using quantitative information helps to convey information about progress. For example, I use pain scales and measurement of ranges of motion to quantify results. I also ask patients to estimate their percentage of improvement. In some cases I will read back what patients said on the initial visit using quotes on some occasions. For example:

Could you estimate your percentage of improvement since we started? If there is no improvement, that would be zero percent, if you feel you are half-way to full healing, that would be 50 percent and so on.

It is important to state this in your own estimation. It is also important to know that it is okay to state that you haven't improved. I find that some people resist this because they want to please their practitioners. Once I receive a statement of improvement from a patient I work to provide positive feedback. For example:

Patient: *I think I am about 30 percent better since we started.*

Doctor: *That's wonderful, you are really doing everything necessary to heal well.*

This simple exchange includes positive feedback and lets patients know that healing is ultimately under their control. It sounds simple, but it is surprising how many reports I receive from patients about practitioners who never provide feedback. For example, when a patient with high blood pressure visited her doctor, the nurse recorded her blood pressure and subsequently reported it in the chart. The doctor entered and said something like "Your blood pressure looks fine." The patient then asked what it actually was and the doctor had to grab the chart and look it up and report back to the patient. This gave the impression that the doctor never looked at it in the first place! A better method would have been to say "Your blood pressure was so-and-so and this is a 20 percent improvement since the last visit—you are doing great."

You can also practice feedback on your own. Again it is best to quantify your improvement as well as you can in your journal. Keep in mind that the healing process is not linear. In other words, you will usually experience some improvement shortly after beginning a healing program. This is followed by a plateau phase when it seems as though you are stuck with no further improvement. Keep in mind that in order to get off the plateau you must continue to gather and integrate information from various sources. Once enough information is integrated you will move off the plateau.

The nonlinear aspect of healing is much like learning a complex skill. When I learned to play the guitar, I was excited to learn a few chords after a couple of weeks of practicing. After a short while it seemed as though I could not improve any further. I continued to practice, sought out a teacher, and purchased some books (all information sources). After a while longer I did improve again. My improvement continued until reaching another plateau.

I also experience this phenomenon with patients. We will begin treatment and there is usually some improvement right away. Then, the patient may get stuck in his healing upon reaching a plateau. It is important to continue to provide information at this point until improvement begins again. Sometimes using additional sources of information helps to get past the plateau.

Once you are aware of your improvement, you must give yourself credit for improving. You are the one who is healing. A practitioner does not heal you. Practitioners are only information sources; you do the actual healing. You must not give your power to an external source. Use practitioners and substances such as medications and nutrients as information sources to help you heal.

Much of the feedback occurs naturally, for you will be unconsciously attracted to sources of information to help you heal. Once you have achieved a high state of awareness and are in touch with your problem you will be able to trust your intuition about an information source.

Understanding the keys will enable you to tap into a continuous stream of healing information. They provide the foundation for a system of healing available to anyone who is willing to learn to use it. The information is available at any time and any place. It is there for you whenever you need it.

CHAPTER 4

MAKING HEALING RELATIONSHIPS RESONATE

I am not the best tennis player I know. Most of my forehand shots make it over the net but get to the other side with varying amounts of velocity. This happens despite my attempting to hit each shot in exactly the same way. Occasionally I am successful at hitting a good shot either crosscourt or down the line. When this happens I can actually *feel* it in the racket. The shot feels effortless and the ball moves faster and straighter. It looks simple when watching a professional play, but any of you who have tried making consistent shots can understand how difficult it actually is.

What I experience when hitting a winning shot is a perfect transfer of energy from the racket to the ball. The racket seems like an extension of my arm and the shot feels easy. Energy flows best when two systems are matched, that is, when the strength of the source matches the resistance of the receiver. If the tennis racket is swung too weakly or the ball hits the wrong spot on the racket, the ball falls into the net. Even if I swing as hard as I can, the ball can still have less speed if it does not strike the racket's sweet spot. I, the racket, and the ball constitute a system of sorts. The source of energy is my arm swing, and the receiver the ball. When source and receiver are matched in just the right way we say the system is resonating.

We can apply the concept of resonance to the transfer of healing information. In order to achieve resonance the strength of the information source must match the receptiveness of the receiver.

A few years ago I attended an indoor concert held in one of the oldest venues in the city. The performer was a rock guitarist and I was a longtime fan. I was looking forward to the event and had even purchased the CD beforehand so I could get the most out of the experience. The opening act consisted of an acoustic guitarist who sang modern folksongs. The notes rang out in the large wooden hall and the words were well understood. The acoustics were surprisingly good, given the age of the building.

Then it was time for the main act. After a short setup period the musicians took to the stage and began the opening song. I could barely recognize the tune even though I had listened to the CD many times. It sounded like a muddled mess! It was very loud, but not understandable. A feeling of disappointment came over me. Here we were, the band playing their hearts out and the audience intent on listening but the message of the music could not get through.

I suffered through the first few songs and then decided to head home. As I made my way out of the auditorium and passed through the exit doors I was struck with the dramatic change in the sound. Here I could hear everything clearly and the band sounded just like the CD. I was amazed at how different it sounded with a decrease in the volume. From now on I always carry earplugs when attending concerts. In some cases the earplugs have made a tremendous difference in my hearing the music.

The source was the band, the receiver the audience, and the informational message the music. The first musician was a solo act with an acoustic guitar. The audience could hear him because the volume at which he played matched the space of the hall. The musical message could get through to the audience. The main act was an entire band that played much louder. They overpowered the space, resulting in a poor transfer of musical information.

All of the information sources must resonate as much as possible with the receiver. If the source is too strong it will overpower the system to the point of causing adverse effects. An example would be taking a strong medication that produces many side effects. Likewise, if the source is too weak, then not enough information flows to be effective. The same effect results from modalities such as ultrasound and electrical muscle stimulation. If the stimulus is too weak the electrical or sound signal will not get through the tissue. If too strong it can cause damage. Any time we attempt to transfer healing information we must consider the strength of the source and the receptiveness of the receiver.

Resonating with a Healer

Many times the source of healing information is another person, a healer. In this case it is important for healer and patient to match as closely as possible. Some healers are very adept at working to "match" a patient. It is an actual part of the treatment as the healer takes some time to get "in synch" or resonate with the patient. It is believed that the treatment will be more effective this way.

In order to achieve resonance, one of two things must occur. Either the healer resonates with the patient or both resonate using a common medium. In some healing traditions sounds are used as a medium to facilitate resonance. For example, a healer may use drums struck at a specific frequency similar to the frequency of the brain's alpha waves. The brain produces alpha waves during states of deep relaxation. These alpha waves resonate at a frequency of seven to twelve cycles per second. [1]

The result is a synchronizing of the healer's and patient's brain waves, which facilitates the transfer of healing information. This frequency also happens to be the same as the Schuman frequency, which is the frequency of the Earth's electromagnetic field. The healer, patient, and Earth all resonate together to maximize the flow of healing information.

Music can also be used to achieve a state of resonance. Religions use sounds and music to focus the mind during prayer, producing resonance. The chant of a mantra or the hymn of a choir can unify the singular voices into one whole to create a connection to a higher power.

It is no wonder that music is rich in information. Not only does it contain information in the printed notes but complex information is also contained in its expression. Music is a product of the complexity of human thought. It represents a high degree of information density. Music is very powerful in that it can excite the emotions or calm the nerves. Music can help to achieve resonance as well as act as an information source. In this case, the mechanical vibrations of sound in air convey the information.

I have found that the more I work to resonate with a patient the less I need to do to treat them. For example, early on in practice I would often treat patients by performing several chiropractic adjustments along with a number of modalities such as deep-tissue massage, ultrasound, hot packs, and electrical muscle stimulation. In many cases I overpowered patients with this sort of treatment and sometimes they actually became worse. As I learned more about resonance I did less and less with much better results. My treatment now flows much better and sometimes I only need to do just one adjustment to a key area.

Busy, overbooked practitioners may find it difficult to take the time to practice resonance. The idea of resonance may conjure up visions of meditating or chanting. However, it can be practiced in a very simple way. You can begin by just being in the present moment with someone. Giving someone your complete attention helps to get you in synch with that person. They will sense this and open up to give you more information about their problem. Once you do this you can use other techniques as well to help resonance. These include attention, nonjudgment, honesty, empathy, and caring. All of these help you to make a connection to another. They help to bring you both into focus. Not only will this help to bring about a better solution to the problem, but it also helps to open a powerful healing channel between you both. You will both be, in a quantum sense, entangled.

Entanglement is a relationship between two things. In quantum physics two particles are entangled if they are in some way related to one another. In this case your connection to another constitutes entanglement. We will see in the next chapter how entanglement helps to open a nonlocal channel through which healing information flows.

Attention

You may have had the experience of visiting a busy practitioner. Many times busy practitioners find it difficult to really focus on patients. I personally have been to a number of doctors who were not really present in the moment with me. Some seemed to be in constant motion, with the goal of just getting to the next patient. They did not really listen to my complaints and some did not even give me a chance to speak.

The information about my concerns was reduced to a scribble on a chart and passed to another health-care worker who was also busy attending to too many patients. Talk about losing information! I often felt sorry for those poor souls who spent time in hospitals, their lives reduced to notes on a chart. Perhaps a more holistic way of transferring information could be developed for large hospitals.

During a treatment session your practitioner should focus her or his attention on you. Distractions such as lack of eye contact, phone calls, pagers, and interruptions from staff weaken the connection and reduce the flow of information. A distracted practitioner will send the message that these other items are more important than your problem and take away from the focus of healing.

A distracted practitioner can miss important information about your problem. A large amount of communication occurs through nonverbal channels. It could be that there is much more to your problem than is communicated in sound bites.

Nonjudgment

You may sense that your practitioner has preconceived or present-time judgments about you. This also works against information flow. Practitioners must be as nonjudgmental as possible when delivering treatments. Sometimes practitioners realize that a patient has contributed to his illness through his own behaviors. A patient may not be following the prescribed treatment or may be engaging in destructive behaviors. Or, a patient may have what is perceived as an irritating personality or work in a profession that the practitioner interprets as negative. There are many ways in which we judge others.

Judgment inhibits the flow of healing information. Your practitioner must have an open mind when dealing with patients, working to create a safe environment by being as nonjudgmental as possible. People respond to this by opening up and revealing more important information that can be helpful.

Honesty

Your practitioner should be as honest as possible. Honesty in a professional relationship can be difficult at times as it can be interpreted in a way that crosses professional boundaries. However, it can also be powerful in opening up a healing channel. Your practitioner can share the emotional experience with you much like a family member or close friend. Honesty is also necessary in providing treatment. Practitioners must fully believe in their treatments. If practitioners provide a treatment that they do not believe in just because a patient thinks it is important, the treatment will be weakened by lack of honesty. In these situations it is better for practitioners to express their feelings about the treatments or make referrals to others.

Signs of a lack of honesty include rote, template-like statements such as "I understand your pain." Your practitioner must be centered in honesty to maximize the experience with you and open up a good informational healing channel.

Empathy

Your practitioner should listen to you with empathy. I have found empathy to be extremely powerful in some cases. Sometimes I have felt that all that was needed was for someone to listen with empathy. Some people have spouses or family members who deny their problem or perhaps even other practitioners who say the problem is "all in their head." Some practitioners have difficulty with this, especially in a busy practice. However, it is an extremely important part of the treatment and your practitioner should take steps to allow enough time to really listen to you.

Most practitioners enter their respective fields because they care about people and want to help. It is amazing how patients can pick up on the effect of a practitioner. They sense that a practitioner doesn't care about them, even if the practitioner puts up a good "front" and acts like she or he cares. Sometimes practitioners enter a healing field because they do care and want to help, but after years of stressful practice, the caring is lost. Perhaps they have not led balanced lives or have let greed be their centers. Perhaps they have even lost what attracted them to healing in the first place. You cannot give what you do not already have. You cannot effectively communicate healing information if that is not your purpose.

It is important not only for the practitioner and patient to match, but that they also select the appropriate information-carrying modality to help facilitate healing. In other words, the team of healer and patient must select the best treatment or combination of treatments for a particular problem. The right treatment will allow more information transfer because it is met with less resistance. The mind can have a powerful effect on healing, especially when the patient has lost belief in the effectiveness of the treatment.

Doubt and Healing

One thing that interferes with resonance is doubt. Doubt about the information source will negatively affect information flow. Doubt will manifest when you feel that your practitioner is too busy to listen to your concerns, or recommends a treatment you do not believe in.

Therefore, you must believe in your practitioner. Choose one because you believe in her or his abilities, credibility, or mode of treatment. People very quickly make up their minds about whether someone can help or not. I have experienced the full spectrum of responses from those who believed I could help them to those who were very doubtful of my abilities. There were even some patients who believed I could help them even though I knew I could not! On the other hand, there were patients I knew I could help but who would not allow it.

Generally, you should have a deep feeling that what your practitioner is doing will help you. If you do not, then the doubt about it will cause interference in the transfer of healing information.

Treatments are also information sources and can evoke doubt. If you do not believe that a nutritional substance, therapy, or medication will help, the healing process will be inhibited. Using practitioners who work to resonate with you will help remove doubt and interference in the healing process.

Simple Exercises to Facilitate Resonance

Here are two simple exercises for practicing resonance. The first exercise will help you to focus on the present. This is important when connecting to a source of healing information, as in receiving a treatment. If you are a practitioner you may be the source of information; thus being in the present with patients will help the flow of information.

Next is a communication exercise using a technique known as active listening. This exercise really helps people to connect when having a conversation. I use this technique a lot in my practice and continually work to improve it. I find that it facilitates communication on a deep level, often helping me to get at the root of a problem.

Learning these new skills may require some practice before getting results. Often there are many opportunities to practice them every day. You only need to be aware of when to do so.

Exercise 1: Being in the Present Moment

There is a Zen story about a monk being chased by a tiger. He jumps off a cliff and is hanging by a vine, a raging river far below. He sees a mouse beginning to gnaw at the vine. Just then he notices a plant with one ripe strawberry. He eats it and enjoys the wonderful flavor. The moral of the story is, of course, to live in the present moment. Our monk can enjoy the delicious strawberry in spite of his impending doom.

We only have control over what happens in the present. Thoughts of the past or future take energy from what is needed for the present. The following exercise will help you to focus on the present.

Take a sheet of paper and divide it into three sections. Label the sections past, present, and future. The sheet of paper can represent one hour or one day. Take a few moments to reflect on your thoughts for that time period, then write them down in the appropriate section of the paper. Think about the amount of energy associated with each thought. Now put a line through all of the thoughts in the past and future sections. These represent wasted energy. Now look at the thoughts in the present section. Put a line through all of the thoughts about things over which you have no control. More wasted energy. What is left are thoughts related to the present. Now estimate the percentage of time you spend thinking about the past and future. For example if you have three thoughts listed in the past section, three in the present, and three in the future you can surmise that you spend more than half of your time thinking about the past and future. Once you are aware of this you can use the following techniques to focus on the present.

1. *Let unnecessary thoughts go. When past or future thoughts enter your mind, work on consciously letting them go. Be aware of them, then let them dissipate. Do not give them energy by allowing them to persist.*

2. *If you need to think about something that happened in the past or will happen in the future, allow a finite amount of time to do so. For example, you could say that you will spend the next hour planning something or working through some past event.*

3. *Don't allow others to control your time and don't fill your time just to do so. Learn how to get out of unwanted conversations. Avoid distractions, especially if you are in a healing profession. Cell phones, pagers, and computers are all examples of distractions. Again, make a limited amount of time for these.*

Just as in learning any new skill, being in the present requires practice. After a while you will notice the benefits of being in the moment. Your day will flow with greater ease. Practitioners will find that patients may respond better. Patients will experience a deeper connection to their practitioners. This will be accompanied by a sense of calm and flow with your surroundings.

Exercise 2: Active Listening

In order to get in touch with what others are saying, you can use active listening. Active listening involves getting at the underlying feelings of the other person and reflecting them back. The listener is present with the speaker and does not make judgments about what is said. The listener simply reflects back his interpretation of how the speaker feels. Active listening is a great example of impedance matching, and when it is done properly, information flows readily.

Use the following guidelines to practice active listening.

- *Really listen to the speaker. Quiet your mind and avoid thinking about what you wish to say next.*

- *Listen without judging the speaker. The focus is on understanding, not problem solving.*

- *Reflect back how you think the speaker feels. Continue to do so until she or he acknowledges that you understand.*

- *Make eye contact.*

- *Nod and shake your head to acknowledge points the speaker has made.*
- *Mirror the speaker's body language.*

The following conversation will help you to use active listening. A list of responses follows the statement. Choose the responses that represent active listening.

> *Jenny is concerned about her stomach pain. She states, "Doctor, I have had this constant stomachache for the past two weeks. I think there is something terribly wrong with me."*

1. Don't worry, Jenny, it is probably nothing serious.
2. We need to run some tests to find out what is wrong.
3. I sense that you feel worried about your pain.
4. Is the pain worse after you eat?
5. I hear some anxiety in your voice.

The active listening statements are numbers three and five. Some people tend to function in the problem-solving mode. Sometimes we are rushed and need to obtain as much information as possible to solve a problem. In healing, the problem is that the disease is seen as something separate from the person. The problem-solving approach tends to work against resonance.

A lack of understanding on an emotional level can lead to doubt. I have seen this many times in my practice. For example, a patient came to me who was recently diagnosed with fibromyalgia by a medical specialist. She was obviously emotionally concerned about her problem. She said her doctor performed the examination and rendered the diagnosis in a matter-of-fact manner. He pulled out a pre-written prescription and handed her a pamphlet. She was upset that her complex set of problems was reduced to essentially two pieces of paper. The entire visit including the exam lasted about ten minutes! As a result of the way he handled her problem, she came to my office looking for help. She obviously had doubts about her doctor even though, in my opinion, he had rendered an appropriate diagnosis and treatment. A little resonance would probably have made the difference in this case.

We can apply the concept of resonance to all of the healing channels in order to maximize the flow of healing information. The way we do this depends on the source. For example, if you are using molecular or energy sources you must consider the dose or strength of the source. Resonating with nonlocal and mind-body sources occurs when getting in touch with the source. This is accomplished with a variety of techniques that will be presented in later chapters.

CHAPTER 5

THE MYSTERIOUS NONLOCAL CHANNEL

When I first graduated from professional school, my head was full of analytical information, and I wasn't afraid to use it. When I look back, I'm sure that my patients absorbed about 1 percent of what I was saying!

After a few years of using this rather mechanistic approach to practicing I underwent a transformation, a paradigm shift. The instructors at my college spoke about healing consciousness and vitalism, but it was difficult to embrace these concepts. How can one use techniques for which there is no measurable explanation? I remember when the transformation first occurred. I was working with a large volume of patients and was really in the moment, or as others would say, "in the zone."

I have had similar experiences where it seemed as if everything flowed. I was moving from patient to patient when somehow I decided to let go of my analytical side and just treat them. With every patient I held a healing intention. I basically stopped the incessant analysis and just became a vehicle of healing information. It was like stepping aside and letting a greater power guide me. My treatments became simpler and my explanations to patients more clear. Many of the daily struggles subsided and I felt less fatigued after a long day.

What I experienced was the flow of information through the nonlocal channel. Information flowed from the information field to me and to my patients. Many practitioners in the healing arts have experienced similar transformations in which they transcended the mechanics of their professions. What could possibly be at work here? Could it be that informational connections exist beyond the mechanistic realm? Can mere intention heal?

We will see that intention indeed plays an important role in healing. Our intentions act as sources of healing information. The information travels instantaneously through what is known as the nonlocal channel. The entire process has an aura of mystery about it. It defies logic and the laws of physics. A few brave scientists have explored this strange phenomenon of nonlocality. We thank them for doing so, for their contributions have opened up a whole new frontier of thought.

Local and Nonlocal Events

Imagine standing with an outstretched arm holding a ball. You drop the ball and watch it fall from your hand and hit the floor. What you have observed is a local event. Local events are described in terms of classical physics, meaning we can use the laws of classical physics to describe the event. Most of the everyday events we observe are considered local. In the case of our ball we can calculate the potential energy in the starting position, the velocity at which it fell, the distance it covered, and so on. All of these calculations are neatly performed with classical physics.

However, let's say this time you again drop the ball, but now you observe a very strange event. Instead of watching the ball fall to the ground, you see it appear on the ground instantaneously. One moment it is in your hand, the next it is on the ground. There is nothing in between. The ball is either in your hand or on the ground.

What you have observed is a nonlocal event. Nonlocal events have very strange properties, not explained by classical physics. Considering that you kept your eye on the ball at all times, the ball must have moved faster than the speed of light in order to get to the ground so quickly. According to classical physics, nothing can move faster than the speed of light.

Nonlocal events have three distinguishing characteristics. They do not carry a signal or propagate a force through a medium. They do not decrease in strength over varying distances. Lastly, for an event to occur in classical physics there must be a start and end time. The event occurs along a time continuum. Nonlocal events occur instantaneously, an impossibility in classical physics. The time interval in a nonlocal event appears to be infinitely small.

The Nonlocal Transmission of Information

Healing information can flow through a nonlocal channel. A number of healing techniques encompass nonlocality, including Reiki, homeopathy, and prayer. Some healers say there is a transmission of healing energy. The problem is that no one has been able to detect or measure any energy. There may be a minute amount of energy or energy of an unknown type that may be measured in the future. Or perhaps there is no energy at all. It may be that healers are capable of transmitting pure information.

It seems as though once two people form a relationship they also somehow form a connection. It is like making a phone call to another person. You dial the number and hear the other person's voice. There is a physical connection between both of you. The connection could be in the form of wires or microwaves. The same thing happens when you relate to another person. This connection, however, is not a physical connection. The connection occurs on a quantum level. Your relationship to another constitutes what is known in quantum physics as *entanglement*.

Once two people become entangled in a quantum sense they may be capable of transferring information nonlocally. Entanglement is one of the mysterious phenomena of quantum physics. The concept of entanglement was developed as an answer to a potential paradox put forth by Albert Einstein in order to disprove quantum physics.

Einstein could not fully accept quantum physics for quite some time. In fact, quantum physics and Einstein's own theory of relativity do not fit together. They seem to contradict each other. Einstein thought that quantum physics was wrong, particularly the idea that we live in a universe wrought with probabilities—thus his famous quote, "God does not play dice" with the universe.

Einstein wanted to disprove quantum physics so he, along with Boris Podolski and Nathan Rosen, came up with a paradox in 1935 known as the EPR thought experiment. Their idea was to create a two-particle pair from the same source so that if one particle is spinning one way, say to the right, the other spins to the left.

Once the particles are created they are sent off over a large distance. Let's say particle A is sent to Washington, D.C. and particle B to Sydney, Australia (a fair distance). We measure particle A in Washington and find that it spins to the right—now we instantaneously know that particle B is spinning to the left. Before we measured particle A, the probability of either particle spinning right or left was 50 percent. After measuring particle A in Washington, we know with certainty the direction of spin of particle B. How did particle B, in Sydney, know the result of the experiment in Washington?

Einstein knew that nothing could travel faster than the speed of light. Therefore if one of the particles somehow communicated with the other, the message could not travel faster than light. And yet the information seemed to travel instantaneously between the particles. Einstein knew this to be impossible and had much trouble accepting this.

One of the discoverers of quantum physics, Niels Bohr, described the results of the EPR thought experiment in terms of a *relationship* between the two particles and an observer. The three were somehow linked and formed a system. It was said that the particles were *entangled*.

In 1964, physicist John Bell devised an ingenious experiment to test Einstein's proposal. Bell developed a theorem for describing the strength of this relationship between particles. Bell's theorem inspired a number of experiments. The results of these experiments supported Bohr's explanation of the EPR experiment. In other words, once the particles were related (entangled) they were somehow able to communicate with each other.

Particles such as those in the EPR thought experiment exist in what is known as indeterminate states. That is, they exist in multiple states at the same time. We said that particle A may be spinning either to the right or left. This is actually not a true statement because, according to quantum physics, the particle is actually spinning in both directions at the same time! It has the *potential* to spin in either direction but begins by spinning in both directions. That is, until consciousness enters the picture. Once consciousness observes the particle, the indeterminate state ceases to exist. Consciousness somehow chooses which state it will exist in. In our case, the particle will then either be spinning to the right or to the left.

Quantum physics tells us that there is such a connection between matter and consciousness. This connection allows for the instantaneous transmission of information. In other words, the information is transmitted nonlocally. Consciousness plays a very important role in providing meaning to the universe. Consciousness is not only our connection to the physical world, but also somehow defines it.

If consciousness is somehow connected to physical events, then how does this information travel? Or what does it travel through? These are tough questions with no concrete answers. However, two researchers discovered some clues. Experiments conducted by Alain Aspect and Nicolas Gisin in the 1980s and 1990s demonstrated that the speed of the information transfer between particles was much faster than the speed of light. Aspect and Gisin's experiment resulted in a speed of 20,000 times faster than the speed of light![1] It appears as though the particles are connected in some way so that there is a nearly instantaneous communication of information.

It has also recently been shown that if a third particle is entangled with one of the original pair of particles and encoded with information, then when one of the particles is measured along with the third particle, the remaining particle somehow transforms into the quantum state of the third particle. This means that information can be nearly instantaneously transmitted to one of the particles. Physicists call this *quantum teleportation*.

An article by Dr. Larry Dossey points out an important implication of the connection between consciousness and matter. He states if particles existed before consciousness, what state were they in? If the existence of consciousness is required to observe waves, then one could surmise that without consciousness there are no waves. He goes on to say:

> *The waves and the electric and magnetic forces…are part of our efforts to understand this mechanism and picture it to ourselves. Before man appeared on the scene, there were neither waves nor electric nor magnetic forces; these were not made by God, but by Huygens, Fresnel, Faraday and Maxwell.*[2]

Dossey's statement implies that consciousness has the ability to change the physical world. This of course would have to occur within the framework of the laws of the physical world. For example, you could not use consciousness to open doors—at least this would be an improbable event. All events may be possible but some are very improbable. Another implication is that matter exists in indeterminate states until observed. The universe is a set of possibilities, with certain possibilities manifesting once observed. If we look at this in terms of information, we see that the universe contains a large amount of information that is not in a contextual form.

According to physicist David Bohm, there is a field of what is known as potentially active information everywhere. Bohm's information field is analogous to the zero-point field.[3] Consciousness activates this information. Consciousness puts information into contextual form; it gives it meaning.

Nonlocal Communication Between People

Can people form relationships that enable them to send nonlocal information to each other? Can this information be used to heal? The answer to these questions seems to be yes. Actually, there is a considerable amount of research supporting this. Much of this research involves people affecting outputs of machines known as random event generators or REGs. These carefully designed machines are capable of producing a random stream of numbers. If a human being can change the output of a REG by simply thinking about it, then there must be some connection between the human and the REG.

Building a truly random machine is no easy task, especially one that produces randomness from quantum events. Helmut Schmidt built such a machine.[4] He used the decay of a radioactive isotope (strontium-90) as the source of random events. The decay of radioactive elements is a random process. As the isotope decays, it emits an electron. The emission of an electron cannot be predicted and it is a truly random event.

Schmidt connected the isotope to a counter that continuously sped through a loop of numbers between one and four. As electrons were emitted from the isotope they struck a detector that stopped the counter. Four lights represented the counter's output. When an electron struck the counter, one of the four lights would light. Because of the randomness, no one could accurately predict which light would turn on next.

A participant would have a 25 percent chance of selecting the next light according to chance. Any deviation from chance would indicate that somehow the participant had affected the machine. Schmidt wanted as strong an effect as possible so he decided to use people who felt that they were able to transmit information nonlocally. Schmidt decided to use psychics to test his hypothesis. He conducted many trials and found the success rate to be 27 percent instead of the 25 percent predicted by chance.

At first glance this may seem like a rather paltry effect. Possibly the results indicated an error, but in the statistical world if the effect holds up to statistical testing it is considered a strong effect. Schmidt's results held up to rigorous statistical testing. The data did indeed show that subjects had some sort of effect on the machine. [5]

Schmidt's early studies using REGs caught the interest of more researchers, including Robert Jahn, founder of the Princeton Engineering Anomalies Research center (PEAR). Robert Jahn is a physicist whose work in such areas as plasma dynamics and aeronautical engineering is highly regarded. Jahn first became involved in REG studies through the work of a graduate student he supervised. The student provided a good case for research into the human-machine connection, and Jahn decided to pursue this type of research. He partnered with psychologist Brenda Dunne to conduct a number of studies on the mind-machine connection.

They developed their own REG using an electronic random noise generator rather than an isotope to produce random events. Their REG produced binary numbers (ones and zeros). The subjects sat in front of the machine and attempted to influence it by willing the machine to produce more ones than zeros, followed by another trial of producing more zeros than ones. This type of design allowed for a large number of trials. They also used a more sophisticated statistical test to analyze their data, looking for deviations from the mean in a data set.

After the first round of trials Jahn and Dunne analyzed the data. What they found would be hard for any rational researcher to believe. The data showed a neat distribution that shifted to the right in one trial and shifted to the left in another. They literally had hard scientific proof that the subjects influenced the machines! The subjects were in some way able to connect with the REGs and change the output.[6]

These initial results spawned many subsequent studies with new REGs in various settings. PEAR team member Roger E. Nelson did a tally of all of the research on REGs. According to Nelson, 108 subjects have performed 1,262 experimental replications consisting of 5.6 million trials investigating this phenomenon. Other variables in these experiments included individual differences among subjects, location of subjects, type of random source, type of feedback, length of runs, and changes in effect over time.[7]

The results of these experiments showed a strong relationship between intention and the output of random event generators. This constitutes strong scientific evidence that humans can affect machines through intention. The research also showed that the effect was larger for two cooperating subjects and for bonded couples, and was not diminished by distance. The effect was larger still for groups having a "unifying thematic or ceremonial aspect."[8] In other words, it is the relationship between people that entangles them.

But does everyone have this ability equally? A study conducted by a team consisting of Cindy Crawford, Wayne Jonas (a medical doctor), Roger Nelson, and Margaret and Mietek Wirkus examined the differences in REGs set up in a library and in a healing practice.

Wirkus is an internationally known healer from Poland who uses healing energy to treat patients. His treatment primarily consists of fifteen-minute sessions in which he conducts an initial scan of the patient followed by sending bioenergy to the areas in need. The team set up a REG in the treatment room and another as a control in a library five miles away. The two REGs were carefully calibrated with each other by using the data from one million trials. The two REGs had to produce exactly the same statistical data set.

The research team was careful to control for such variables as temperature and the attention Wirkus might have given to the REG. Three experiments were conducted at different times. Basically, these consisted of turning on the REG thirty minutes before the healing session and letting it run for thirty minutes afterward. The idea was that the REG would deviate from statistically neutral results during the healing sessions. When a REG deviates from neutral, it is known as an anomaly. So the researchers were looking for a greater number of anomalies during healing sessions, as compared to the control REG in the library.

What they found was that the REG in. Wirkus' office did indeed produce more anomalies than the library REG. On average the REG in the office produced 34 percent more anomalies than the REG in the library. The result was statistically significant and cannot be accounted for by chance. There was a definite effect produced by the healer. The researchers interpreted the results of this experiment as the same result of all REG research:

> One explanation invokes a process whereby HI (healing intention) actively reduces disorder (entropy) in the environment. The concept is that engaging in a healing encounter alters the degree of disorder in the space associated with that encounter, resulting in increased order and homeostasis for the patients.[9]

Other research has investigated the effects of healing intention on bacterial growth,[10] wound healing in mice,[11] and skin conduction.[12] Some experiments investigated the experience of a subject's awareness that he is being stared at. In all these studies it appears that the strength of the effect from person to person is stronger than that from person to machine.

The Nonlocal Channel

What is common to all the above research is that people have the ability to decrease randomness in another person or machine. Randomness decreases with the addition of information. All the research points to the idea that people can transfer information nonlocally. But exactly how does such a miraculous transfer occur?

It seems as though no conventional explanation exists for such events. When scientists attempt to either find or measure energy, they usually come up empty handed. Energy cannot be responsible for these anomalies since energy must obey the laws of physics and cannot travel faster than the speed of light. Energy transfer cannot explain an instantaneous transfer of information. Also, energy diminishes with distance. If energy were responsible, the strength of the effect would decrease with distance. Again, this is not what happens. The strength of the effect does not seem to depend on distance.

A theory regarding the transfer of information developed by researchers Jahn and Dunne describes information exchange between individuals as occurring in a connected system.[13] When an individual is part of a system, the conscious identity of the individual is decreased as the individual connects with the system. This is much like being a member of a group. The members of the group are related in some way. For example many churches encourage their congregations to pray for members who have become ill. The members form a relationship in which each member loses some of his personal identity to that of the group. In a quantum sense the members are entangled; they are related in some way. The relationships among group members decrease the entropy of the group. The group becomes less random with these connections. Since these connections are established, it is easier for the members of the group to send nonlocal healing information.

People can send information nonlocally and the ability to do so improves when they form relationships with one another. Consciousness allows for the transmission of nonlocal information through its ability to make choices. Consciousness then must move in a direction to choose. It must have some kind of purpose; it must have an intention.

Intention is very powerful with regard to information exchange. Consciousness works through our intentions to affect the physical universe. However, intention is a two-way street. Our intentions can help us to heal or hurt us. They can make our lives easier or much more difficult. As the old adage states: "Be careful what you wish for…"

Healing Intention

Healing intention encompasses the transmission of healing information through a nonlocal channel. When I decided to incorporate healing intention into my practice, my patients improved. Healing intention is an extremely important aspect of healing. Our consciousness is continuously receptive to receiving new information. It also seeks what is needed. If someone is in need of healing and is receptive to information exchange, then consciousness will seek the information needed to heal. This is such an important concept that I believe all practitioners should incorporate healing intention into their treatments.

Consciousness gives meaning to our lives. Your individual consciousness through intention is always seeking, always gathering information from its surroundings to put into context, to provide meaning. There are unlimited possible states of existence. Your consciousness chooses among these states.

So why then do we do the things we do? Why do some of us continue to follow dysfunctional patterns of behavior, attract the same kinds of people into our lives, and end up with the same results? The answer lies partly in our genetics and neurophysiology, and partly in our intentions. Our brains establish neural patterns from the beginning of our existence. Some of our behaviors are wired at birth with tendencies to behave in certain ways inherited from our families. The more these behaviors are performed, the stronger the neural connections become, and the more difficult it becomes to change them.

So how do we change these patterns? Many psychology textbooks have been written about this, but we are interested here in the idea of information. Therefore, one way is by acquiring information. Information provides a framework for a contextual shift. The context in which we perceive events, our understanding of the world, changes with the addition of new information. We have all experienced this. We have a distinct view of something, then learn something new about it and have an entirely different view.

The key is to be aware that there is something to learn and to approach it with an open mind, bearing no judgment. Let consciousness seek information in its purest form, guided by our intention to heal, unclouded by previously conceived notions, with empathy and with understanding. When this approach is taken, the universe provides unlimited information.

Awareness is the first step toward a perceptual shift. We must be aware that a shift can occur and be aware of our role in creating our present thought patterns. Once we become aware, the channel opens for information to flow into our consciousness. Thus as we learn about our illnesses and better understand our role in the disease process we are better able to change it.

On the other hand, if we refuse to accept our role in disease or deny its existence, our consciousness works to support the disease. You may have experienced this with someone you know. This is the person who, for some reason, wants to hold on to their disease. Perhaps they have been playing the victim for years and the disease lends credence to their self-perception. Perhaps they use their disease to manipulate others, or to obtain sympathy and benefits from those around them. Some even go so far as to define themselves in terms of their disease. Little do they realize that their actions actually work to support the disease.

Using healing intention is a very powerful way to transmit or receive nonlocal information. Healing information flows with intention. Intention is an important piece of the healing puzzle and can be used in conjunction with any healing modality.

CHAPTER 6

USING THE NONLOCAL CHANNEL

Imagine the power of sending healing information to anyone, anytime, anywhere. You can actually do this using the nonlocal information channel. In the previous chapter we saw that everything is connected in a field of information. A change in one part of the field causes an instantaneous change elsewhere in the field.

There are two primary skills we will be concerned with when using the nonlocal channel. The first is connecting to the information field; the second is receiving and sending healing information through intention.

I found these skills of immense value in my own healing. They were a bit difficult to practice at first, but eventually became part of my life and continue to be today. They gave me direction and allowed me to remain on a healing path, to stay the course through the hard times. You see, there were times when I did not think I would heal. I would experience a setback and get discouraged. The old symptoms and behavior patterns would return. Sometimes I would lose the intention to heal and just try to again cover up the symptoms with medication, distractions, and work. Initially having the intention to heal is relatively easy; maintaining it through years of an illness can be very difficult.

I have such a strong belief in nonlocal healing that I think all healing should begin this way. It does not require a lot of time and effort, but it does require being consistent.

Connecting with Meditation

Probably the most used and studied technique for making a connection to the information field is meditation. There are a number of forms of meditation and we will examine just a few. Meditation can be done by anyone and is fairly easy. You need only a willingness to do it and a quiet place.

Consciousness is continuously working to put information into context. Our link to consciousness is through our minds. Since much of the information we receive comes from the external world, our minds can become distracted with numerous thoughts from external sources. In meditation we turn our minds inward as we decrease the amount of external stimuli. Meditation quiets the mind while still maintaining awareness.

Meditation has been studied extensively, starting with the work of Herbert Benson, MD, a Harvard researcher and author of the book *The Relaxation Response*.[1] Dr. Benson's work was the first formal research on meditation in the Western world. His work linked meditation to many physiological and psychological benefits. Many subsequent studies have supported and added to Benson's research.

One form of meditation called TM, short for transcendental meditation, was introduced to the Western world by Maharishi Mahesh Yogi in 1959. In the 1960s TM gained popularity when a number of celebrities including the Beatles learned and practiced the technique. Since then, millions more have learned to meditate, and there is now university in the Maharishi's name. According to Maharishi University, there have been over 500 studies supporting the efficacy of meditation.[2] Many contemporary clinics and hospitals teach meditation as a powerful stress-management technique.

A fascinating study in the *Journal of Crime and Justice* reported that crime rates were lowered when a group of people meditated in a sample of cities. The original study was performed in eleven cities and was later expanded to forty-eight with similar results. The study was controlled using other cities of similar population characteristics and crime rates. It appears that a community of minds functioning together in a common cause can influence the minds of others in a nonlocal way.[3]

Meditation Techniques

The first technique we will describe is called *mindfulness meditation,* which is derived from the Buddhist tradition known as *vipassana,* in which one focuses on the present moment.

Mindfulness is an introspective state in which thoughts are observed and noted but no analysis or action is taken. To begin, find a comfortable (but not too comfortable) position such as in a chair. The classic posture for meditation is sitting cross-legged in the lotus position, but it is not necessary to do so if it is uncomfortable. An upright posture helps by supporting your spine. The idea is to be comfortable but not sleepy. You will be working on getting into a state of increased awareness, so you must not fall asleep. The area should be as free from distractions as possible.

Once you are in the right position, close your eyes or relax them so they are partially closed. Start by quieting your mind using deep breathing (see page 102). Then focus your attention on an object, word, or phrase for a few minutes. At this point you are ready to begin practicing mindfulness. When thoughts enter your mind, just note and observe them, but take no action.

An important thing happens when practicing mindfulness: you begin to live in the present moment. It is surprising how much of the day we spend not doing so. We spend a lot of time thinking about where we need to go or what we need to do in the future. Maintaining a busy schedule, thinking about getting to work or going home or the weekend are all instances of living in the future. Similarly, we spend time thinking about the past as well. Constantly thinking about a problem we need to solve is a good example of not being in the present moment.

Directing conscious attention to the future or past produces noise in the nonlocal information channel. Mindfulness helps to reduce this noise and allows information to flow in. It lets you step out of your mind and observe your thoughts. Doing so allows an increased awareness of the present moment, as well as a deeper perspective on and understanding of your thoughts.

As thoughts come into your mind it is important not to engage in any analysis or reaction to them. Instead, you need to accept them because that is what is happening at the present moment. Mindfulness is not an escape from reality; it is a fuller experience of reality. When you experience reality on a deeper level you are better able to deal with it.

For example, if you are using mindfulness as part of a healing program and you are feeling sick or in pain, it is important to accept these sensations so that you can deal with them more fully. In mindfulness, you must try not to escape the pain or sickness. You must go with the sensations.

You can practice mindfulness meditation at any time. You could set aside a certain time of the day that is free of distraction or you can just check in and be mindful throughout the day. After some practice, it becomes easier to achieve a mindful state. In my own experience, I frequently found my mind wandering when seeing patients. In a busy practice it is difficult to stay on schedule since some patients require more time than is scheduled for them. I found it most difficult to be mindful during these busy times, for I could hear the waiting room become more crowded in the background. It took much practice to become able to take small segments of time to really focus on the present moment.

I especially enjoy practicing mindfulness during exercise. One of the components of my exercise routine is to walk on a treadmill. The repetitive nature of this activity helps me to maintain a mindful state. I have had similar experiences with riding a bicycle or walking. The combination of mindfulness and endorphins really creates a state of calmness.

Simple Breathing Meditation

This simple exercise can be done nearly anytime. The exercise incorporates diaphragmatic breathing and mindfulness meditation. To begin, you need to find a distraction-free location where you can be comfortable sitting. Noisy environments can also work if you are able to tune out the ambient noise. With practice you will be able to meditate nearly anywhere.

Once you are comfortable, close your eyes slightly and focus on your breathing. Be aware of how you are breathing, especially how your breath begins. Your breath should begin with your stomach moving outward. Your stomach should move out and then your chest should slightly rise at the end of your in-breath. If you find yourself initiating your breath from your shoulders, work to relax them. Notice the rate of your breathing. You should be taking slow, regular breaths.

Continue to focus on your breathing, initiating each breath with your stomach. Clear your mind of distracting thoughts. If you start to think of something besides your breathing, just return your attention to the breathing. You can acknowledge thoughts as they enter your mind but work to let them go. Do not linger on any particular thought.

Focused Meditation

Another form of meditation centers on focusing on an object, word, sound, or phrase for a given length of time. This is done after getting into a relaxed state by using focused deep breathing or progressive muscle relaxation. Again the object of the exercise is to be relaxed, but to remain alert. After achieving a relaxed state, you clear your mind and focus on the object. If other thoughts enter your mind you must let them go and return your focus to the object.

This type of meditation also requires practice. At first focusing your attention may be quite difficult, and you may feel restless and unable to control the thoughts that continually enter your mind. If you have difficulty with this, start with brief periods and then gradually increase the time as you gain proficiency with the technique.

Active Meditation

Engaging in certain activities can also induce a meditative state. Playing an instrument, painting, or just taking a walk are examples. The mind becomes quiet when engaged in creative thought. It is as if the actions come from another source than your own mind. Creative activities can be useful in a healing program.

Painting or playing an instrument can become an actual part of the healing process and an expression of feelings associated with healing. Not only is your mind quietly producing a state of creativity, but your inner thoughts and feelings are expressed through the creative act. It is important to do such activities in a truly creative way and to avoid left-brained or logical thought as much as possible. For example, if you are playing an instrument, do not focus on intense reading of music but just play whatever comes to mind.

Meditation can bring about a more relaxed and calm state of being. With regular practice you will improve your skill so that you can meditate virtually anywhere. You may feel a deeper connection to everything around you as well as to a higher consciousness. Meditation works to open a nonlocal channel to the information field by reducing noise so that your intention to heal can focus your mind and connect with consciousness. Your intention to heal provides a deep purpose, a deep meaning to your life. Once all of the extraneous noise is eliminated your purpose comes through. Consciousness makes the connection and information flows. Many of us can sense this connection. I describe it is as a deep knowing. When I was ill and was forced to deal with my physical problems, I carried with me a deep knowing that somehow I would eventually overcome my illness. Others have described it as a deep sense of security or a peak experience where everything flowed without resistance.

Intention

As we saw in the previous chapter, healing intention is one of the most important forms of nonlocal communication. Healing intention is simply the practice of performing activities with the purpose of healing. A sick person can have the intent to heal her- or himself, or a practitioner can have the intent to heal a patient.

Intention and motivation are intimately linked. Motivation can come from two primary origins. You may be either internally or externally motivated. Motivation can be explained in psychological terms as what is called *locus of control*. Locus of control is based on the social learning theory of Julian Rotter.

Locus of control has to do with the perception of control in your life. If you operate from an internal locus of control you are internally motivated; that is, your life is controlled by your needs, desires, and actions. If you operate from an external locus of control you are externally motivated—meaning your life is controlled by other people or situations.

Rotter saw people as motivated by positive stimulation. In other words, people will naturally seek out positive stimulation and avoid the negative. He also described the personality as intimately connected to the environment. One cannot separate the two. If one wishes to change personality, then one must either change the environment or change one's thoughts.[4]

Personality is not a static entity but is dynamic and changing, since it continually takes in information resulting in change. This is analogous to a student taking a course to learn new material. The student may begin with a certain set of beliefs that change as learning progresses.

Internally motivated people see themselves as responsible for whether or not they gain positive feedback. Externally motivated people see outside forces or events as responsible for feedback. Internally motivated people may determine that their behaviors contributed to their becoming sick, whereas externally motivated people see outside influences as responsible.

Let's look at two fictitious people, Mary and Joe. Both became ill with the flu. Mary has an internal locus of control while Joe has an external locus of control. When questioned about why she became ill, Mary responded with answers such as:

> *"I must not have had enough sleep the last few days."*
>
> *"I have been working too hard lately."*
>
> *"I have not been washing my hands as much as I should during the flu season."*

Joe responded:

> *"The flu always happens to me around this time of year."*
>
> *"My wife was ill and she gave it to me."*
>
> *"My coworkers were sick and gave it to me."*

Those who are internally motivated seem to cope better with disease. They take responsibility for their role in the process and have more control over it. By being internally motivated, Mary has a much greater chance of affecting outcomes.

Those who are more externally motivated tend to hold others such as doctors or family members responsible for their disease. Some externally motivated people see disease as a chance event. They were just "unlucky" to have contracted an illness. Or it was "their time" to become ill. Externally motivated individuals have much less control over their disease process. In fact, a "victim" mentality can lead to an increased incidence of disease.

Why would internal versus external motivation be important in having the intention to heal? Internally motivated individuals express intention more powerfully. Externally motivated individuals see intention or purpose as an external event. External motivation inhibits connections to the nonlocal information field, because the motivation does not occur at the core of the individual. The intention must be consistent with the purpose of the individual. The individual, at their core, must want to heal.

Practicing Healing Intention

People practice healing intention every time they act with the purpose of healing. Healing intention occurs anytime someone visits a doctor or other healing practitioner, takes a medication, or engages in any other healing activity. The connection exists in these activities; what is needed is to strengthen and maximize this connection.

To help maximize the connection, if you tend to be externally motivated, you must work on becoming more internally motivated. You can do this by performing some introspective work, investigating just what your actual purpose is. The intensity of the work depends on just how externally motivated you are. In the extreme case people try to prove their doctors wrong by remaining ill or becoming worse. Some people identify so much with their illness that they resist any movement toward health. The result is a frustrating situation for family members, practitioners, and anyone else wanting to help. The person's inner thoughts seem to be saying something like:

> *I guess I will try this new technique, but I know it will not work or will even make me worse!*

The first step in becoming more internally motivated is to take responsibility for your problem. It may be that your actions have directly contributed to the problem or it may be that they have not. In either case, your present state is in some way a result of your thinking and actions. To help you become more internally motivated, ask yourself the following questions and deeply contemplate the answers.

What is my role in my problem?

What actions of mine have contributed to my problem?

What actions of mine have contributed to my life situation at present?

What have I done to heal myself?

Can I see myself improving?

Do I think that my actions will affect my improvement?

Am I focused on healing?

Do I feel empowered in my healing?

Do I use other sources of information to complement my healing?

When your intention to heal is powerful, you will be rewarded with moving toward healing. When giving power to others or events clouds your intention then there will be interference with healing. The stronger your intention to heal, the stronger you connect to the information field.

Healing Intention for Practitioners

The following section is for practitioners wishing to use healing intention in their practice. Nonpractitioners will also find this section useful in evaluating practitioners.

Any practitioner of any healing art can use healing intention. It is very simple to use on a daily basis with any patient. All it requires is being in the present moment with the patient and focusing on the connection to the information field with the intent to heal. It sounds easy, but sometimes it can be a challenge—especially if you see many patients or your office is full of distractions.

To use healing intention during a visit, all you need to do is follow these steps:

1. Be present with the patient.
2. Take a moment to connect with the information field.
3. Allow the information to flow through you to the patient.

Being Present

This step does not have to take much time. It can be as brief or lengthy as you wish. Of course you should always be present with patients when they are communicating with you. This means keeping distractions to a minimum. This can be quite difficult if you are not used to it. As many patients come and go throughout the day, it is easy to get caught up in the "mechanics" of your practice. Logically solving problems here, directing the staff there, taking phone calls from patients, vendors, other practitioners all take your attention away from patients.

I had to work hard on this concept myself. As my practice grew, so did the daily demands on my time and energy. At one point I likened my role in the practice to a "plate spinner." The plate spinner is a circus performer who keeps a large number of plates spinning on sticks. He starts off with a small number of plates, then adds them one by one until there is an unbelievable number. All the while he runs from plate to plate not allowing one to hit the ground. I found it hard to focus completely on the patient because I always had the feeling that one of the plates was about to fall!

After changing my scheduling process, getting rid of my pager, and informing my staff not to interrupt me when I was seeing patients, I was able to focus more on patients and be in the present moment with them. This allowed me to work on healing intention. I always felt that I did a better job when I performed healing intention, and in fact my results improved dramatically. Not only did more patients heal, but also new patients were attracted to my clinic.

Connecting to the Information Field

Once you are able to practice being in the present moment you can move to the next step. This connection is a very personal thing and you must work on developing your own method. I can give you some techniques to help and you can modify these to your own liking. When you are at peace and centered the connection is easy. If you are distracted, in pain, or ill, the connection becomes more difficult.

To make a connection you must quiet your inner mind much as in the technique of mindfulness meditation described earlier. You can then form an image of healing information flowing through you to the patient, recite a short prayer, or do both. The method of getting into this state does not matter. It is the *intention* that matters. In my practice I always allow some time for physically touching the patient;

since I primarily work with patients with musculoskeletal problems I always need to palpate the problem. This gives me the opportunity to practice healing intention by centering myself, using imagery, and reciting a brief statement.

Letting the Information Flow

The image I use is that of a light originating from above and flowing through me, through my hands and into the patient. When I establish this image of a connection I recite the following statement:

> *Divine light flowing through me,*
> *Bless this patient and allow them to heal.*

The entire process takes but a few seconds. I always feel a sense of calm and connection to the patient. You can use the above statement or develop your own. It does not matter—it is the intention to heal that matters. If you are a more visual person you may develop your own image of healing or if you're a more touching person, focus on the feeling of healing.

Since this kind of information transfer occurs nonlocally, it is necessary to practice it in the presence of the patient. The instantaneous transfer of information can occur anywhere, anytime. For example, you could just center yourself and think about a patient healing. Healing information can be transferred this way.

Sometimes I have thought about a patient who discontinued care, but was not healed. It might have been months or years since they came to see me. I would focus on the person and would receive a deep knowing that they would return to complete their healing. Many times they called the very same day. I have spoken to numerous practitioners about this phenomenon and they have had similar experiences. If patients need what you can offer, their consciousness will attract them to you.

The exercise outlined in figure 6.1 will help you develop your own healing intention. It is best to take some time to reflect before developing your intention. When you are ready, write it down and let it be your guide in your healing process. When you follow the process of

Writing Your Own Healing Intention

If you are in need of healing, you can develop your own healing intention. Use the following guidelines:

- Write your intention in the present—for example, a statement such as "I am healing" or "My pain is lessened." Statements such as "I will heal" or "My pain will go away" are written in the future.
- Use definite statements such as "I know that I am healing every day," or "I know that my pain is diminishing."
- Acknowledge your connection to the universal source of information.
- Show gratitude.
- Conclude with a definitive statement about your healing.

Here is an example:

I know that every day I am healing. I know that as I go through life I accept what I need to heal. My illness decreases every day as my body gains strength. I know that this is so because the universe provides what I need to heal and I am connected to it. I know that this is the truth and I am grateful.

Example for fibromyalgia:

The pain in my muscles is fading away every day. My connection to the universe is providing what I need to heal and my body accepts it. I feel new energy as my pain diminishes. I am thankful that I am healing. I know the information I receive every moment directs my path away from pain. I know that this is so.

Example for high blood pressure:

I feel relaxed as blood flows smoothly through my body. I see the blood flowing through the relaxed vessels of my body. I know the universe provides the information I need to heal. I accept this with gratitude and I know that this is the truth.

Healing intention for a Practitioner

I am here to transfer healing information to my patients. I am thankful that I can be a part of their healing. I know that we are all connected and our connections can be used to give what is needed for healing. I know that there is truth in what I am doing.

It is best to focus inward when writing or saying your healing intention. Remember that the mind integrates this information and changes to provide what is needed. It is best to have a period in your day in which you relax or meditate if only for a few moments and then state your intention. It helps to repeat your intention at least once per day. Our minds need to be reminded. If you are a practitioner you will find a greater sense of purpose. If you are a patient you will discover a greater sense of control over your health.

Figure 6.1 Writing Your Own Healing Intention

writing your intention, your reality will change. You will gain control over your health and become more focused on healing. Let your intention guide your healing.

CHAPTER 7

THE MIND-BODY CHANNEL

M any times I have wondered if what I was doing with my patients really helped them to heal. There were times when I administered what I thought was the perfect treatment that resulted in things becoming worse and there were times when I did practically nothing and the patient improved. I have witnessed numerous patients with the same diagnosis—some who improved, others who did not. I often pondered why this was so. I have witnessed patients who suffered from arthritis pain who became enthused about a new nutritional supplement and reported that they were feeling great and pain-free, only to have the effect eventually wear off and the old pain return. This phenomenon occurred after events such as trying a marvelous new exercise or a fantastic new herbal remedy, a magic bracelet purchased at a flea market, or just seeing a great new doctor. It was as if their belief in the remedy produced the healing. As their belief wore off, so did the healing effect.

This next information channel can be used by anyone to send healing information to the body. In chapters five and six we saw that our minds can connect with consciousness. Now we will see how powerful the mind is as a source of information to the body. The channel is the mind-body channel. The mind is the source, the body the receiver. The information is carried by the neuroendocrine system with its complex connections to every system of the body. Since our minds serve as an information source, much depends on our perception, beliefs, and even our interpretation of the world in which we live. What we think has a profound effect on our physiology.

Your mind is an informational structure. Consider your brain and its vast number of interconnecting cells, called neurons. Your brain contains over one billion neurons. Connections are made and reinforced through experience. As your brain receives information from the senses, it forms new connections or strengthens old ones. Each neuron communicates with other neurons by sending tiny packets of chemicals called neurotransmitters. This extremely complex structure communicates with the rest of your body in two basic ways. Either neurons secrete neurotransmitters directly into organs or the brain secretes other chemicals called hormones that travel via the bloodstream to the various tissues of the body. The secretion of hormones and neurotransmitters collectively is called the neuroendocrine system. Every part of the body is somehow affected by the neuroendocrine system.

Voodoo, Witchcraft, and Hypnosis

Many traditional healing systems were aware of the mind's effect on the body. The mind's role in healing was an important part of the healing process. These systems frequently included the use of altered states of consciousness to facilitate healing.

Some of the most powerful effects were seen in cases of voodoo and witchcraft. Witch doctors exerted extreme power over their subjects by casting spells and using herbal remedies, both thought to be inert. The word *voodoo* comes from the African word for spirit. It was the spirits (called *Loa*) in voodoo that held the power to affect lives. These spirits are still worshipped today in the Vodun religion practiced in Haiti, Benin, Ghana, Togo, and the Dominican Republic. Vodun is also practiced in areas where Haitians have settled.

Since the spirits held the power, they were worshipped in rituals held for various reasons including healing. Vodun rituals began with a feast, followed by beating drums, shaking rattles, and chanting. Dancing to the rhythmic beating and chanting continued until the Loa possessed the person. The ceremony concluded with animal sacrifice as the spirits were appeased. It was believed that these rituals allowed contact with the spirit world. The spirits could exert great power over mortal lives.

Although most Vodun priests practiced their religion for good intentions, a few practiced what was known as black magic. One technique employed by such priests used a doll representing a person— the proverbial voodoo doll. The priest would stick pins in the doll to curse the unfortunate soul. Voodoo, at its most powerful, could produce great healing—or its opposite, death.

The power of the witch doctor or Vodun priest was contained in the power of suggestion. Curses transmitted negative information to an unfortunate person in the form of a suggestion. The recipient's negative perception of the curse was able to produce powerful negative effects on his or her body. The power of voodoo, like all mind-body phenomena, lies in the perception and beliefs of the subject.

Mind-body healing was not restricted to traditional systems such as voodoo. It found some recognition in the medical profession in the late 1800s, when the famous hypnotist Jean-Martin Charcot worked with patients suffering from psychosomatic illness. In one of Charcot's dramatic demonstrations, a patient with hysterical paralysis could walk while in a hypnotic trance. Hypnosis was found to be beneficial in treating other ailments as well. Patients with emotional disorders, asthma, and dermatitis also experienced positive responses with hypnosis.

The use of hypnosis continues today in less dramatic fashion to help with a variety of psychological problems such as anxiety, smoking, weight loss, and overcoming phobias. Some athletes find that hypnosis helps them perform under pressure.

Jerry the Skater

I became interested in the mind-body connection during my study of psychology as an undergraduate. Sports psychology was an emerging field at the time and one of the goals of the field was to improve performance using mind-body techniques. One of my research paper assignments was a on how the mind affects human performance. I decided to use a case study of an athlete, a figure skater named Jerry.

Jerry was preparing for a skating test in front of a panel of three judges. In order to pass he was required to skate a routine set to music. The routine had to include a number of difficult jumps and spins. Jerry seemed ready and had worked hard at preparing for the competition. He could consistently perform all of the maneuvers in the program. He could also perform the program two times back to back without missing an element. Jerry had the intention and ability to complete his program and pass the test.

I decided to frame this situation as if it were an experiment, so I looked for potentially confounding variables, factors that could interfere with Jerry's performance by changing between the warm-up and the actual test. According to my observations, everything looked consistent: the ice surface, temperature, people observing, and noise level. Even Jerry's skates were exactly the same between the warm-up just before the test and the actual test. It was also interesting that the judges watched the warm-up so Jerry was actually performing in front of them.

During the warm-up Jerry performed all of the elements of his program in front of the judges flawlessly. He warmed up for as long as he wished and when he felt ready he signaled the judges. He took his position on the ice and the program music started. He appeared confident and in control as he started to move across the ice. He skated into his first difficult maneuver, a double jump that required him to land on one foot without the other touching the ice. He skated into the jump and proceeded to go out of position and miss the timing, which resulted in a fall. He got up and continued. I had observed Jerry fall in practice before and he was able to recover and complete his program on many occasions. All was not lost at this point because there were a number of other maneuvers to be performed and he still could pass the test.

He skated into his second jump with a look of determination on his face. I could tell that he was working hard not to repeat the same error. But on the second jump he again missed his timing and fell. After that the rest of the program was a disaster with multiple falls.

Jerry came off the ice devastated and confused. I was at a loss for an explanation myself. Everyone appeared disappointed. A few minutes later the test chairman delivered the unwanted but expected news that Jerry had failed the test. Jerry just sat there thinking about what had happened.

I have witnessed this phenomenon at countless sporting events. Athletes who were obviously capable of performing well could not do so when it counted. I have also heard this from many students in my classes. What they experience is commonly known as *test anxiety*. In test anxiety, the nervous system interferes with performance.

In Jerry's case everything was exactly the same between his warm-up and the actual test. The only thing that was different was what was going on in Jerry's mind. Jerry had *doubted* his ability to perform. His belief that he could perform the program was shaken at the moment when it counted. His mind changed the physiology of his body to the point of making him unable to do what he had been doing for months.

There is a physiological explanation for what happened to Jerry. It has to do with a part of the nervous system called the autonomic nervous system (ANS). There are two parts of the ANS, the sympathetic (SNS) and parasympathetic (PNS) nervous systems. The SNS tends to cause excitation and the PNS tends to calm things down. For example, the SNS causes an increase in heart rate, blood pressure, and breathing. The PNS has the opposite response.

Both systems work together to maintain balance in the body. Jerry's problem was that his doubt manifested in fear. The fear activated the SNS, which in turn sent signals throughout his body that interfered with his performance.

Since then, when observing sporting events, I always watch for doubt emerging in one of the players or teams. Sometimes you can see it in the faces of team members who have just fallen behind in the score. Other times it emerges as tentativeness in a skill. Sometimes doubt is what makes the difference in very close contests. When players or teams are equally matched, the presence of doubt is enough to decide the winner—the reason athletes who perform at a high level constantly work to minimize doubt about their performance.

In the same way that doubt can cause problems in performance, it can also cause problems with healing.

The Informational Explanation

How can voodoo, witchcraft, hypnosis, fear, and doubt be explained in terms of information? What was the informational mechanism that caused Jerry to fall apart when it counted?

We have learned that all living beings require a constant supply of information in order to survive. Since our senses are bombarded with information from a variety of sources, it is up to the mind to sort through all of this input and put the information into context, to somehow give it meaning. To heal, the mind must take this information and use it to reduce entropy in the body.

We are blessed with marvelous and powerful minds that are capable of moving us toward either health or illness. Our minds are tremendous information processors that have equally tremendous control over our material bodies. We only need to point our minds in the right direction.

Nobel laureate Gerald M. Edelman describes a model of consciousness in which the mind is seen in terms of information processing.[1] Edelman sees the mind as a system capable of selecting information that makes a difference to the system from a larger set of information.

The selection process decreases the randomness (entropy) of information. The mind puts the information into context, giving it meaning. As information is organized into contextual form, the entropy decreases.

According to Edelman, in order to achieve conscious awareness, the mind must exhibit a certain degree of complexity. The level of consciousness or arousal is a function of this complexity. The more complex the mind becomes, the higher the levels of consciousness that are possible. As we have seen in previous chapters, life itself evolves to more complex levels. As the complexity of life increases, so does consciousness and so does the mind.

This means that as information is integrated into the mind it becomes a more complex informational structure. The increasing complexity of the mind influences the decisions it makes.

The mind continuously attempts to make sense of its existence as it strives to put information into context. A simple example would be to observe a random arrangement of spots of various colors on a white page. Although there is virtually no information to be gained by such an observation, the mind will attempt to find a pattern or organization to the arrangement of spots. If you asked a series of observers what they saw in such an arrangement you would get a variety of answers. One observer may see the face of someone famous, another a familiar object, and so forth. The mind tries to make sense of the display by providing a context for the spots.

The act of putting information into contextual form can be thought of as activating information by bringing it into physical existence. Pure information consists of possibilities that have not yet manifested in reality. The information in the mind is in the realm of ideas. The mind can take this information and bring it into the physical world.

The mind does this by making decisions. Decisions can be thought of as *information in action*. Decisions work to reduce randomness, moving our lives in a specific direction. The more decisions are made to move in a specific direction, the more entropy is reduced, and the more likely it is that a path will unfold. Decisions can be conscious or unconscious. Some are made after much contemplation while others are automatic, seemingly springing forth from our deepest being. We may even have an inborn tendency to make certain types of decisions.

We could conjecture that on some level Jerry decided to fail. He may have not consciously *wanted* to fail, but his mind somehow made the decision for him. His decision to fail may have been buried deep in his unconscious mind. He may not have even been aware of it. It surfaced as doubt, which manifested as fear, which in turn triggered his autonomic nervous system to interfere with his performance.

The same process is at work with voodoo and witchcraft. On some level the unfortunate subject's mind *decides* to become ill or even die. The mind takes the information presented to it, interprets it, and gives it meaning. It then puts this information into action by making a decision, sometimes with catastrophic results.

Decisions are of the utmost importance in healing. They can be of immense help in moving us along a healing path. They can also be a roadblock and extremely detrimental to our health. All healing begins with one ultimate decision of the utmost importance that we all must make in order to move in a direction of health. *We all must begin our healing by simply deciding to heal.*

This sounds simple, but in reality it can be very difficult. We still have our unconscious minds to deal with. Jerry may have consciously decided to skate well enough to pass his test, but his unconscious mind was working against him. We typically do not consciously do things that are unhealthy, but we may do so because our unconscious mind is in control. Our unconscious mind may have its own agenda. It may be working to fulfill some deep-seated unhealthy need such as the need to be a victim or the need to control everything.

To begin your healing you must make the decision to heal and take it seriously. I recommend writing it down, as this helps to bring it out of the world of ideas and into the material world. Your decision to heal is closely linked to your intention to heal, as described in chapters five and six. In fact your decision to heal precedes your intention to heal. If you have completed the exercise in chapter six you have already decided to heal.

In informational healing, decision, and intention work two ways. The mind is the link between consciousness and the physical body (see figure 7.1). Thus the mind can connect with consciousness to transfer nonlocal information, and since it is an informational structure in its own right, it communicates with the body via the mind-body channel. Your decision to heal leads to your intention to heal. Once your mind integrates decision and intention, healing information will flow from consciousness to your body.

Now that you have made the decision to heal you must work to get your unconscious mind to move in a direction of health. The techniques in the next chapter will help you do so.

Before we delve into how to get your mind to help you heal, I would like to discuss some of the more indirect ways your mind can affect your healing. These are your personality, how you perceive your job, and your opinions.

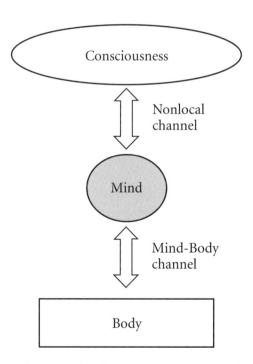

Figure 7.1 Information flows between consciousness, mind, and body.

Personality

Your personality can help or hurt you when it comes to healing. Personality has been linked to health problems such as immune suppression, stress, and heart disease.

It is generally difficult to study personality and disease, since other confounding variables can interfere with the results. The best proof would be to study people before and after a personality change. If the only thing that changed was someone's personality, then the presence of a disease after the change can be more closely associated with the new personality. But how can we study such a dramatic change? How can someone's personality change so rapidly?

Some people do experience such dramatic changes in personality. The most famous of these was Sybil, a woman who purportedly had sixteen personalities. Sybil made multiple personality disorder (MPD) famous. Since her story became public, the diagnosis of MPD skyrocketed from a few reported cases to thousands.

What better way to study the mind-body phenomenon than with people with MPD? The mind, as an information structure, changes instantaneously with the changes in personality. The change in personality results in different decisions made on both conscious and unconscious levels. The decisions are so powerful as to completely change the physiology.

Research by the Institute of Noetic Sciences has shown these extreme changes in physiology in people with MPD. A personality may have a pathological condition such as hypoglycemia or diabetes that will manifest within seconds of that personality emerging. The researchers were able to measure drastic changes in brainwave patterns that occurred within seconds of the personality shift. It appears as though at one instant the mind was sending a certain set of instructions to control the body, then moments later when a new personality emerged, an entirely new set of instructions was sent along, resulting in drastic changes in physiology.[2]

Not only is personality as a whole linked to the physiology of the body, but certain constituents of personality called traits are also linked.

Probably the most famous is the link between the trait known as hostility and heart disease. Hostility is a manifestation of anger. Anger is not only a negative emotion but it can also negatively affect the body's physiology through the mind-body channel. A study conducted by Ted Dembroski of the University of Maryland found that the personality trait of hostility predicted an increased risk of coronary disease.[3] There appears to be a strong link between hostility, anger, and heart disease.

Jodi was a patient of mine whom I had been treating for migraine headaches and neck pain. She was always very animated and had a positive personality. I marveled at how she could juggle the needs of three children, a small business, and a husband who was absent on numerous business trips. The quintessential life of the party, Jodi would also entertain frequently.

I treated Jodi for several years. She would come in on an "as needed" basis when her headaches grew worse in intensity and frequency. I would treat her a few times and they would subside for a while, only to return again in the near future.

After a few years of this I noticed a pattern. For one, the headaches were usually most severe on the weekends following a stressful week. She could endure the stress throughout the week for just so long before it manifested as a migraine. The other thing I noticed was that the headaches increased in frequency around the holidays. It seemed that the additional stress of all the extra holiday tasks such as shopping for gifts and preparing elaborate parties took its toll in the form of headaches.

I eventually came to the conclusion that Jodi had some deep-seated problems under the surface of her seemingly happy existence. Underneath her façade was unhappiness. She was projecting a positive attitude while suppressing her needs. No matter how hard she tried she could not bring herself to meet her needs. Everyone else came first.

It turns out that there may be more than unhappiness under the surface. In fact Jodi may be more susceptible to cancer because of her personality. Researcher Karl Goodkin of Stanford University School of

Medicine, in a meta-analysis of studies of women with a predisposition to cervical cancer, found that women who were self-sacrificing, sociable, overly cooperative, and optimistic to the point of denial were at higher risk for developing cancer.[4]

Dr. Goodkin also found that women who were hostile, fearless, hardheaded, blunt in social situations, and punitive toward others also had a higher risk of contracting cancer. It seems as though these personality traits, taken to extremes, predispose people to the disease. If the traits are kept in check, people are more likely to experience health.

Social Interaction

Besides personality, another psychological factor affecting the mind-body channel is social interaction. We are social beings and social interaction with others seems to be a fundamental need for well-being. If we are isolated or lose social support, say from a loved one, there is a greater risk of contracting an illness. We are all familiar with the concept of separation from a loved one causing a person to become ill or even die.

Research conducted by Steven Schleifer estimates that as many as 20 percent of deaths occurring within the first year of losing a spouse are attributed to factors associated with bereavement. Other research has found significantly increased mortality rates as high as twelve times the norm for married people within the first year of losing a spouse.[5] Social isolation has been related to physiological processes causing decreased immunity and decreased HDL cholesterol, which is important in inhibiting arterial disease.

In general, researchers have found that people who lack social support are less healthy and more prone to all diseases than those who have social support.

Job Satisfaction (Can Your Job Make You Sick?)

We spend a large portion of our waking lives working, so it seems logical that our jobs can have an effect on our physiology. It depends on how we perceive our job. The same job can energize one person while draining another. Many of us have experienced dissatisfaction with job functions, coworkers, and supervisors. Unhappiness stemming from a job can have a profound effect on our lives, but can effects of poor job satisfaction go beyond an unhappy eight hours per day?

Job dissatisfaction was the best predictor for heart attack in a study performed by a task force commissioned by the Department of Health, Education and Welfare in Massachusetts.[6] Job strain is also an important factor in high blood pressure. Research has shown that job strain is also associated with heart problems.[7]

Various factors influence job satisfaction as a whole. These important factors include a sense of control in decision-making and the opportunity for job growth. The factors rely on the perception of the individual. If you are not satisfied with your job because you feel you have little control over decisions made that affect you or are stuck in a position with little or no opportunity for advancement then you may be at increased risk for disease.[8]

On the other hand, positive job factors are associated with good health. Job factors that are positively related to a decrease in potential heart problems appear to fall into three primary categories. First is a sense of control over one's situation in the workplace, such as the opportunity to make decisions regarding work functions. Second is the opportunity for growth and a sense of challenge on the job. Third is having a commitment to work, family, and community.

Our thoughts and perceptions have a powerful influence on our health. Mind and body, thoughts and physiology are intimately linked.

Can Your Opinions Make You Sick?

How healthy you think you are also helps to determine how healthy you actually are. Your perception of your own health is a powerful information source. Research has shown that one's perception of health is a powerful indicator of actual physical health. A series of studies involving 23,000 people found that the opinion of health was better at predicting actual health than medical signs, symptoms, and laboratory tests. [9]

Our beliefs and opinions have a powerful influence on our bodies. If we believe something or someone can help us, then it probably will. My patients who wore the magic bracelet that took away their arthritis pain (at least temporarily) really believed it would do so. Like the Tin Man, Cowardly Lion, and Scarecrow in the *Wizard of Oz* we can elicit power from certain objects and substances. This placebo effect has been studied extensively.

Powerful Placebos

A placebo is an inert substance, the proverbial sugar pill that is incapable of eliciting a physiological response from the body. So its effect depends more on the belief in what will happen than the actual chemistry of the placebo. In medical research the placebo response is treated as a confounding variable, something that interferes with an experiment. A medication is seen as effective if the response to it is greater than the response to a placebo. Some have gone as far as to say that some alternative medicine practitioners are just using the placebo effect to get results. Generally it is seen as something to be discounted, an effect that has no mechanism or is not based in reality.

In fact, the placebo response is present in many healing systems— including conventional medications. In Ernest Lawrence Rossi's landmark book, *The Psychobiology of Mind-Body Healing*, he states:

> *There is a remarkably consistent degree of placebo response, averaging about 55 percent of the therapeutic effect for all the analgesic drugs studied. That is, while morphine obviously has more potent analgesic effects than aspirin, about 55 percent of the potency of each is a placebo response.*[10]

And:

There may be a 55 percent placebo response in many, if not all, healing procedures. Such a consistent degree of placebo response also suggests there is a common, underlying mechanism of process that accounts for mind-body communication and healing, regardless of the problem, symptom, or disease.[11]

These are very powerful statements. They imply that about half of the effect of virtually any treatment is due to placebo. Or to put it another way, about one-half the effect of any treatment is due to the belief that one will improve. This is such an important concept that I believe all practitioners should work to facilitate the placebo response. I do not support the idea of giving sugar pills to patients, but I do believe in supporting the belief that they will heal. We will explore ways to do this in future chapters.

Just how can an inert substance such as a sugar pill promote healing? It has to do with how the mind perceives the placebo. The mind interprets the placebo in the context of healing. Once this is done the mind *makes the decision to heal.* Healing information then flows from the mind to the body via the neuroendocrine system.

Although placebos are seen as inert substances in the physical realm, they can be very powerful in the realm of the mind. Some people respond to placebos better than others. Certain personality traits can either facilitate or interfere with healing. The traits associated with a good response to placebos include:

- Being more subjective than objective
- Believing in their practitioner
- Creativity
- Flexibility

Such an individual is capable of using more right-brained processing than left. The right side of the brain processes information of a subjective nature while the left side is more analytical. The right side is more nonverbal than the left. The right side processes information in a more holistic fashion and the left in a more linear way.

Artists and musicians often rely on right-brain thought processes to produce creative works. In fact, many times logical or linear thought processes inhibit creativity. Creative works seem to originate from a different source than logical thought. Perhaps the creative mind reaches deeper into the subconscious than the analytical mind.

It may be necessary at times to let go of analytical thinking to allow mind-body healing. Sometimes we use logical thought to talk ourselves out of something. We must keep an open mind when it comes to healing, as some things work on levels of which we are unaware.

We must allow our minds to work with us and not against us. I am convinced that the mind is motivated to seek healing information on a deep level. Illness sets the mind in motion to locate the information necessary to heal. We need to get in touch with this deep motivation to allow the process to flow without roadblocks.

CHAPTER 8

USING THE MIND-BODY CHANNEL

Mind-body healing is an important part of any healing program especially when dealing with the more severe illnesses such as cancer. Anyone can use the mind-body channel for any illness. All it takes is a little time and patience. This chapter is devoted to helping you use the mind-body channel in your own healing. Here you will find a variety of techniques designed to activate your own mind-body channel. The techniques are seemingly simple, but can elicit powerful results.

Opening the Mind-Body Channel

Brain scans (PET scans) have shown that when a person thinks about performing a certain activity the same sections of the brain are active as when the actual activity is performed. In sports psychology, athletes rehearse performances by getting into a relaxed state and going through a successful performance in their minds. Muscle activity has also been measured when a person concentrates on performing a maneuver. Concentrating on a performance causes activity in the same muscles used in the performance.

To illustrate how the mind-body channel works, try this simple experiment. You will need a piece of thread, a button, and a sheet of paper with the design in figure 8.1. Tie the button on to the thread so it dangles at the end of the thread.

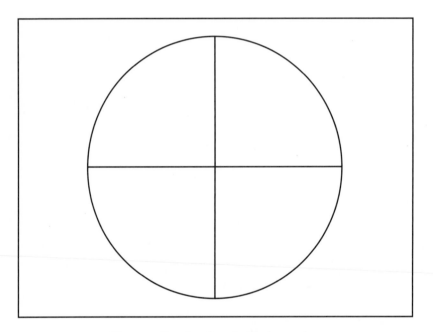

Figure 8.1 Template for mind-body exercise.

Place the paper on a table and sit facing it with the elbow of your dominant hand resting on the table near the design. Flex your wrist in a relaxed manner and hold the thread with the button with your thumb and first finger so it dangles over the design. Let the button come to rest just over the center of the design. Now without consciously moving your hand, just think about the button moving back and forth along one of the lines. Before long it should begin to move just as you think it should. Now think about the button moving along the other line. Again it is important that you do not consciously move your hand or fingers. The button appears to move just by thinking about the movement. Now get creative and move the button in a circle, first clockwise then counterclockwise. You may even be able to get the button to move in a figure-eight pattern. All of the movements are controlled by your mind.

Of course what happens is that the mind sends information to the muscles of the fingers and hand to move the button. However, you do not need to consciously move any of the muscles in order to move the button. It all happens automatically.

Here is another example designed to produce a physiological response through use of the mind-body channel.

Close your eyes and get into a relaxed state. Clear your mind of any distracting thoughts. Now, with your eyes closed, hold both arms straight out in front of you. Visualize that attached to your right wrist is a string connected to a large balloon. Concentrate on the lightness of the balloon and feel the pulling on your wrist. Feel the balloon float up toward the sky. Now visualize that attached to your left wrist is another string connected to a heavy weight. Feel the weight pull on your wrist toward the earth as it gets heavier and heavier. Focus on these images for a few moments, then open your eyes and look at the position of your arms. If you were successful in opening a strong channel, then your arms should be separated by a significant amount.

Decide to Heal

In the last chapter we saw how the mind works to put information into context by making decisions. We said that decisions represent information in action and work to reduce entropy by adding information to a system. Before beginning mind-body healing, or any healing, for that matter, you must consciously make a decision to heal.

Making this decision helps to focus your mind on healing. It works to give you permission to heal and avoid negative influences. It also provides a starting point from which to move forward in your healing. Your decision will open your mind to seek healing information from the universe.

It is important to make a declaration to heal and to put your decision on paper. This will bring it out of the world of ideas and into the physical world. It will become something solid instead of theoretical. It will also give you a sense of purpose in your healing.

Once you have done this, you can move into the following mind-body techniques. They are all designed to help focus your mind on providing healing information to your body.

Get Relaxed

Before practicing mind-body healing you must get into a relaxed state, free of distractions. One way to do this is by practicing deep breathing and a muscle relaxation technique such as progressive muscle relaxation. I will describe a technique called *diaphragmatic deep breathing*. Many people breathe primarily with the shoulder and chest muscles. This leads to increased stress and pain in these areas. This kind of breathing generally indicates stress or some kind of guarded state that inhibits breathing. I see many chest breathers in my clinic who suffer from stress and muscle tension. Many times a little practice with proper breathing goes a long way in helping to reduce stress.

The chest breather elevates the chest during the first part of inspiration by activating the shoulder and chest muscles. These muscles are not designed for this kind of repetitive activity and develop stress, tension, and eventually pain. In order to breathe properly, practice the following technique:

> *Lie on your back in a comfortable position, with both hands on your stomach. Now take in a deep breath by pushing your stomach outward as if to make it larger. Feel your stomach move outward with your hands. You will find that the first part of your breath will occur from contraction of the stomach muscles fol-*

lowed by a slight rise of the chest. It is important to initiate the breath with the stomach and then follow through with the chest. If you were to observe yourself breathing you would see a wave starting at the stomach and ending at the chest. Your shoulders should not elevate at any time during the breath. Take a few seconds to exhale, relaxing as the air leaves your lungs. Now consciously practice this a few times. It will eventually occur automatically with practice.

In my opinion the best time to practice deep breathing is before going to sleep at night and when waking in the morning. The idea is to *set* your breathing for the night and for the day before going about your daily activities. You may also wish to check your breathing periodically throughout the day. If your shoulders are elevating, then you are not breathing properly.

Once you are able to breathe properly you can move on to progressive muscle relaxation. The basic technique of progressive muscle relaxation consists of breathing in and holding your breath for about five seconds while tensing a muscle group. You then exhale and relax the muscles while feeling the tension flow out of them. You can start anywhere in your body, but you should get to all of the major muscle groups. You can repeat the exercise as many times as necessary for tight areas. I have found that in many patients the shoulders and neck harbor a lot of tension.

The following is a sample session of progressive muscle relaxation.

Get into a comfortable position, either lying down or sitting in a comfortable chair. Focus on your breathing and take some slow deep breaths with your eyes closed. You may wish to monitor your breaths by putting your hands on your stomach and feeling it move in and out as you breathe slowly and deeply. Try to clear your mind of any distracting thoughts.

Now take in a deep breath and tense the muscles of the feet for about five seconds. Then exhale and relax them, feeling the tension leave the area. Next, focus on the legs. Take in a deep breath, hold it and tense the muscles of the legs. Hold the tension for about five seconds then exhale and let it go, feeling the tension leave your body. Now move on to the stomach muscles...

Continue with the muscles of the chest, back, hands, arms, shoulders, neck, and face. You can be more general by contracting large muscle groups such as both legs at the same time, or more specific by contracting just the back of the right lower leg, then the front, then the back of the left leg, etc.

Progressive muscle relaxation gets better with practice. I remember the first time I tried the technique by listening to a forty-five-minute cassette tape given to me by a practitioner. I did not feel much of a difference after completing the exercise and the tension returned shortly afterward. However, after a few weeks of practice I was able to scan my body to look for tension and reduce it significantly with a few repetitions of tensing and relaxing the muscles.

Once the technique is learned, it is quite useful to use a body scan to help reduce tension throughout the day. To perform the scan, just stop what you are doing at the moment, close your eyes. and scan your body by feeling for areas of tension. If you come across such tight areas, just take a few slow, deep breaths and perform a few contractions and relaxations focusing on the tension leaving your body. Figure 8.2 outlines the 10-step body scan.

I have found the body scan very useful, since a significant amount of my work time is spent in front of a laptop. Some days I am not even aware of the tension growing in my neck and shoulders until a mild headache starts at the base of my skull. However, if I stop and scan the area and perform a few contractions, I feel much better.

Deep breathing and progressive muscle relaxation prepare you for a mind-body healing session by helping to free your mind of distractions and relax your body.

The 10-Step Body Scan

It is surprising how much tension we can hold in our bodies throughout a normal day. Muscles held in a contracted state for long periods of time can cause a variety of problems. Besides robbing the body of energy, contracted muscles can inhibit breathing and form tender, painful areas that inhibit movement.

Sit comfortably, close your eyes and direct your awareness to the various parts of your body. If you find a tight area, contract the muscles in that area for 3–5 seconds then relax them. Focus on feeling the tension drain out of the muscles. You may start with the following sequence, but as you gain skill in locating your tight spots you can adapt the sequence to fit your needs.

Scan your body in the following sequence:

1. Right leg
2. Left leg
3. Buttocks
4. Abdomen
5. Chest
6. Right arm
7. Left arm
8. Shoulders
9. Neck
10. Face

If you find tight areas contract the muscles as follows:

1. Legs—straighten both legs and point the toes
2. Buttocks—squeeze together
3. Abdomen—draw in the abdomen
4. Chest—bring your shoulders together in front of you
5. Arms—bend elbows and wrists
6. Shoulders—bring shoulders up to ears
7. Neck—bend head forward and then backward
8. Face—scrunch up

Figure 8.2 The 10-Step Body Scan.

Using Imagery

Once you are relaxed you can use the mind-body technique known as imagery. Imagery has been used for thousands of years and can be traced back to ancient religions. Tibetan Buddhists use imagery in prayer, focusing on a deity to invoke healing powers.

Imagery has also been used in the science of psychoneuroimmunology (PNI). PNI is a relatively new discipline that studies mind-body healing. Imagery is but one of many of the techniques used in PNI. Imagery can be done in a clinical setting or alone and has been shown to be effective in alleviating pain and promoting healing.

After achieving a relaxed state. you can begin to visualize your disease or symptoms. It is important to develop a specific image to attach to your problem. Sometimes when focusing on the problem an image surfaces, and other times you must create one. The image may also change periodically. Changing images indicate that you are getting at other aspects of the disease or are healing at a deeper level. Your image must have some meaning to you. The image I used for my heart was that of a red light emanating from my heart. I would then imagine a blue light bathing my entire body, replacing the red light from my heart. I would feel a sense of calmness with my exposure to the light. Other people have used images such as lightning bolts striking cancer cells or shrinking black spots representing tumors.

Once you can image the problem you will concentrate on some method of dissipation. Examples would be making the image dissolve or replacing it with another healing image. I had one patient who visualized a small, troll-like character who smashed the disease with a hammer.

The imagery exercise should be performed once or twice per day. It typically takes about thirty minutes to one hour to go through it. Some find it difficult at first, but it gets less so with practice. It may also take some time for the body to integrate the information sent by the mind. You must exercise patience throughout this process as healing may take some time.

Once prepared, begin to get in touch with the problem or disease by creating an image of it. It is important to develop your own images of the problem, as they are more powerful if they come from your own mind. Sometimes the image is not clear and may be associated with feelings or words. This is perfectly okay. Remember that there is information transfer occurring, and information can exist in words (auditory information) or feelings (kinesthetic information).

Now that you have produced an image of the problem, you need to develop a solution to it. Some people imagine the image of the disease dissolving or breaking up. Others visualize a healing image that overtakes the disease image. Here is an example of an imagery session for low-back pain:

> *Now that you are relaxed and focused, visualize your pain as a bright red ball located in your lower back. As you approach the ball, you feel the discomfort of the disease. It gets stronger as you get closer. Now, imagine a blue healing light. The light enters your body and travels throughout your body. The blue light reaches the ball and enters it. The ball becomes filled with the blue healing light. As the ball fills with the blue light it starts to break up into pieces. The ball breaks up and the pieces dissolve away until nothing is left but the blue healing light.*

Imagery helps to open the mind-body channel so that healing information flows from the mind to the body. Think of using this channel as you would use any other, or like taking a medication. Figure 8.3 outlines the imagery exercise. Use it at least once per day in your healing program.

Some people have difficulty producing images. This is perfectly okay as we are not all equally adept at processing visual information. The basic idea is to produce some entity in the mind that represents the disease, then to somehow manipulate it by either dissolving it or replacing it with another healthy entity. I have had problems with imagery when attending guided imagery sessions with a practitioner. The practitioner would tell us to produce an image of the problem and my mind would go blank! I found it better to do imagery alone in

Developing Your Own Imagery Exercise

1. Create an image of your problem.

It is important to relate your problem to an image or symbol. It may be something like a dark cloud or rays of red light or whatever you wish. What image comes to mind when you think of your problem? Write down a description of your image:

_____

_____

_____

_____

_____

2. Create an image of health.

What image comes to mind when you think of perfect health? Write down a description of your image:

_____

_____

_____

_____

_____

3. Get into a relaxed state.

Sit or lie in a comfortable position. Close your eyes and focus on your breathing. Breathe in slowly by pushing out your stomach muscles for a count of three. Breathe out by relaxing your stomach muscles to a count of three. Do this for a few minutes. During this time try to clear your mind of all thoughts. After you feel relaxed, create the image of your problem in your mind. It is important to make a mental connection between the image and your actual problem. Now imagine replacing the negative image with the positive healthy image. The negative image can be replaced or destroyed by the positive one.

Figure 8.3 Developing your own imagery exercise.

an area free from distraction. Occasionally, my images were not strong visual images but contained some component of feeling.

Imagery may also bring up other aspects of the problem. The process of using imagery allows the mind to go deeper into the problem. This can allow memories and sensations to enter the consciousness. Some people gain a deeper understanding about their problem this way. As the other aspects surface they are to be dealt with one by one. In some cases there are such deep roots to a problem that therapy conducted by a professional is necessary.

Autogenic Relaxation

Another technique used to achieve a relaxed state is called *autogenic relaxation*. This technique is a bit simpler than progressive muscle relaxation and many people find it useful. The basic concept is to first locate a tight area in the body and then focus on it relaxing. You do not need to contract the muscle as in progressive muscle relaxation, just let the muscle relax by concentrating on it.

Autogenic relaxation works well with body scanning once you become practiced in scanning. You can scan your body for tight areas throughout the day and then try to relax them. I have found this technique useful when incorporating it with a posture scan. When the body is in proper alignment, the muscles supporting it naturally relax. I have instructed my patients with postural problems and subsequently chronic tight muscles to use this technique.

Many people sit at desks or use computers for a good portion of their workday. They are not always in the best posture when doing so and this leads to tight muscles, which can lead to myofascial pain syndrome. The idea is that not any one particular posture is that bad; it is the time one is in the posture. For example, throughout my day I sometimes find my shoulders rounding forward and my head tilting downward. This begins to create stress in my neck. To help to counteract this effect, I do a posture scan. Sometimes I get up and take a short walk and focus on maintaining good posture. This helps to take the stress off the neck muscles. I find when I do this the neck muscles naturally relax when I sit down at the computer again. Autogenic relaxation can be made easier with good posture.

Deep breathing intensifies the results of autogenic relaxation especially when deep breathing is performed first. Start by taking a few deep breaths, then scan your body first for posture and then for tight muscles. You may naturally want to stretch first before settling down. After the posture scan, perform a muscle tension scan looking for groups of tight muscles. Then concentrate on those muscles relaxing. Finish with a few deep breaths. You can now begin an imagery exercise.

Putting Your Subconscious Mind to Work

So far we have examined some techniques for getting healing information through the mind-body channel primarily by using the conscious mind. Deep breathing, muscle relaxation, and imagery use conscious thought. To go deeper, the subconscious mind must be brought into the process. The subconscious mind can be accessed from the conscious.

Your subconscious mind is always at work solving problems and putting information into context. Have you ever had the experience of having a problem at work or school and no amount of conscious thought was able to solve it? You may have given up on thinking about it, only to awake one morning with a solution. Many great discoveries were made this way throughout history.

Your Private Mind-Body Session

The first step in getting the subconscious mind to work is to allow it to connect with the illness internally. This can be done with a therapist or alone in a quiet environment. To prepare, use one of the relaxation techniques described above. After you are relaxed you must connect with your illness on a deep level. Perhaps there are memories or feelings associated with the problem. You are encouraged to connect with these. In order to form this connection you must think about your illness. Ask yourself the following questions when doing this exercise. They will help you to connect on a deeper level.

What do I feel besides pain?
Why do I feel this emotion?

Is this emotion connected to something else in my life?

What does my illness mean?

What is the meaning of my pain?

Does my pain have a useful purpose?

Are there any memories associated with my illness?

Once you access the deeper feelings and memories you should just take a few moments to experience them. Keep this time to just a few moments. Next you will explore solutions to your illness. The idea is to get your subconscious mind to work on solving the problem of the illness. You should answer the questions:

What is my role in my illness?

What can I do for myself to help me heal?

This will help your subconscious to do two things. It will work on the problem and stimulate your subconscious mind to seek healing information from the environment. Finally, it is important to visualize what it would be like to exist in a healed state.

The following steps summarize the process:

1. Prepare to engage the subconscious mind

2. Visualize (connect with the problem)

3. Explore solutions

4. Visualize what it would be like to be well (healed state)

This technique may allow other issues to surface that are related to the main problem. These must be dealt with as each one is experienced. For example, if feelings surface they should be experienced, if another problem surfaces a solution should be sought. Sometimes you will gain an insight into your illness. Healing is a process and may require numerous steps that bring you closer to healing.

As you proceed through healing by invoking your subconscious mind, you may experience certain memories associated with your illness. The mind stores information by way of memory, reconstructing an event so that it can be recalled. This process can be triggered and facilitated by sensory stimuli. Certain sights, sounds, or smells can help the brain to reconstruct memories. The information held in memory is dynamic and changing with the infusion of new information—thus memories change as time continues. This means that as you progress through the healing process the memories associated with the problem may change.

It's best to practice this technique for a certain period of time, say thirty minutes to one hour. This is about the same as an imagery session. However, the sessions may vary in length from a few minutes to an hour. It depends on how much the subconscious has to do. Generally, you will achieve a relaxed state; allow your mind to work on the problem and then return to a waking state. When your mind has finished the process you may feel agitated or have a desire to stretch or change position. These are signals that your mind is finished for this particular session.

Once you have started this technique, you may find that things surface in your consciousness such as memories or feelings. You will need to explore these in your private mind-body sessions. These are all part of the process of healing.

I used my subconscious mind many times when working on my own healing. It provided deep insights into my problem. Many things surfaced from these sessions including negative thought processes from my childhood, my ideas about work, and even my faith. I found it very useful to bring these out of the subconscious mind so that I could deal with them.

Engaging Your Illness

You do not need long sessions of mind-body techniques in order to open a mind-body information channel. The following technique simply requires you to engage your illness. This means getting in touch with your illness on a deeper level.

In today's society, many of us tend to ignore our illnesses or try to deny them. This works against healing by inhibiting the mind. We should work to get our minds involved in healing. The mind has such a powerful influence over our bodies that to inhibit it closes off an important healing channel.

A certain television commercial comes to mind when I think of how we deny illness. This commercial is for a long-acting cold medicine. A railroad worker is working outdoors on a cold, wet day. The rain is pouring down and he is soaking wet. He exclaims that when he takes this particular medicine when he has a cold he can keep on working up to twelve hours!

The message here is let's suppress our symptoms so we can continue to stress our bodies. Now our bodies have to deal with the illness, the stress of working, and metabolizing the medication! Instead we should engage our illness in order to understand why we have it or what we can do about it.

One way to engage your illness is to ask yourself a question or series of questions, according to the following framework:

How am I responsible for my illness?

What am I doing to treat my illness?

Is my treatment working?

Taking responsibility and listening to your own answers will help to put your subconscious mind on the right track. You will also have a deep sense that what you are doing is right for your illness.

Practitioners can ask similar questions in a clinical setting. Generally, I present questions in the form of a kind of homework assignment to patients. An example would be:

"I would like to give you a question or two that I want you to really think about for your next visit. I really need this information from you in order to fully understand your problem. For your next visit I would like you to give me three reasons why you have lower back pain."

Patients either write the answers out or tell them to me. I present the questions in a very supportive and non-threatening manner and I give them some time (between visits) to develop the answers. This allows for some processing time between visits. During the subsequent visit they usually have no problem coming up with at least one obvious answer, but my goal is to have them go deeper into their problem. I want them to really reflect on their role in their illness. Doing so enables the mind to work on the problem.

An example of a question with the goal of going deeper would be:

"Can you think of any nonmechanical reasons why you have lower back pain?"

Such questions engage the patient's mind in order to determine their role in their illness. This is one aspect of activating the mind-body channel. The next part involves engaging the mind regarding the treatment via the following questions:

"What do you think your body needs in order to heal?"

"Can you think of three things your body needs to heal?"

"What do you think you can do at home (or work) to help you heal?"

Again, simple questions are followed by a question that goes deeper, such as:

"What can you do to help your healing process besides taking medication?"

"When you've thought about your pain, have any memories come to mind?"

"Do you have any other feelings about your problem besides your pain?"

The final part of this engagement exercise is to provide positive feedback. Acknowledging that patients are on the right track and are healing well can do this. This positively reinforces the engagement process and allows the mind to continue working on the problem. It is quite gratifying to witness the positive change in patients as they progress through this process.

Some people are more accepting of this deeper level of treatment than others. It is important to get help from other professionals if necessary. You can determine whether you need such help by how you feel. If you have problems dealing with what surfaces during this process, seek professional help.

I have referred people to other practitioners when necessary. For example, on some occasions when treating patients with chronic pain a strong psychological component surfaces. In numerous automobile accident cases, I have found that emotions such as fear and anger surface during treatment. Sometimes the feelings are so strong that I need to make a referral to a mental-health practitioner. I generally refer these people to a psychologist who deals primarily with chronic pain issues. I have also found that somatoemotional release techniques are useful for these people. Somatoemotional release is a treatment that addresses the emotions associated with muscular problems. It was developed by Dr. John Upledger and is based on the idea that emotions can be stored in physical trauma.

Feedback

Healing is a process much like learning. Healing and learning both require information exchange. They are both active, dynamic processes. I know that when my students are actively involved in their own learning, they learn much more. The same occurs with healing. To illustrate active versus passive modes of information exchange, let's look at learning in a class setting.

A student takes two classes; the first class is in history, the second in general science. In the history class, the professor's teaching style is to stand in front of the class and lecture for fifty minutes. There is a brief period at the end of the class when students may ask questions, but the professor does not allow questions during the lecture so that the flow of the lecture is not disrupted. The lectures are elegantly presented and each one could be a chapter of a scholarly book. The student, however, finds it difficult to concentrate on the content and must scramble to write down as much information as possible. Her mind is focused on note taking, with little regard for the content.

In her general science class, by contrast, her professor attempts to engage the class by walking around the classroom asking questions. The questions are simple to begin with, then increase in difficulty. About halfway through the class period, the students are divided into groups to complete an activity that reinforces the content just presented.

In which class do you think more information transfer occurred? In the history class, our student was focused on writing down information to be learned later. Even though she was able to write down most of the lecture, there was virtually no feedback. Important points may be misinterpreted or missed completely. She may end up memorizing her notes for the next examination without making the correct connections or putting the information into context.

In the science class, information was presented by getting the students to think of answers to questions. The professor attempted to engage the students by getting them to think. Feedback was given throughout the class period. Students also had the opportunity to practice what was presented in an activity. This provided even more feedback.

Feedback is extremely important in healing. We saw in chapter two that living systems capture information and form feedback loops. This concept is present in any mode of information transfer and healing is no exception. Your mind forms a feedback loop with the information presented to it. Your mind is automatically attracted to information that helps you along the healing process. This information is integrated into your mind, which in turn is stimulated to seek out more information. You are also using feedback in the engagement process when you ask yourself whether your treatment is working.

You must keep an open mind about this process, for it may not seem logical. For example, I see a fair number of patients who are a bit skeptical about chiropractic. Perhaps they or someone they knew had a bad experience. I work very closely with these patients to provide feedback to help them along.

Mind-Body Exercises

There are three exercises presented here that are designed to help you use the mind-body channel. We have already seen the body scan and imagery exercises in figures 8.2 and 8.3. Figure 8.4 illustrates a forgiveness exercise that will help you to let go of negative information you may be carrying about someone or an event. Forgiveness can be an essential element of mind-body healing. Sometimes we get stuck because we hold on to negative thoughts about someone or something. Sometimes we even need to forgive ourselves for past abuse.

These are three of my favorite exercises and I do them often. I use imagery even when sick with a cold or flu and I use the body scan almost daily when working long hours. I have also taught many patients to do these with good results. I hope you will find them useful.

Forgiveness Exercise

Reflecting on and contemplating an illness can bring up negative thoughts such as blame. Some blame themselves or others for their illness. Blame produces noise in the mind-body channel. People may become "stuck" in their healing since they cannot get past the blame.

If blame should surface you must work to forgive whoever or whatever you feel is to blame. To do this it is helpful to write a statement of forgiveness that you either repeat silently or think about whenever blame surfaces.

Start with the statement "I forgive" _____

Then write a statement about what you forgive the object of blame for. Finally, write a statement about moving forward.

Here is an example:

I forgive myself for eating poorly and contributing to my weight and poor health. I forgive my parents for letting me do so as a child. I will not continue to harbor these negative feelings of blame. I need to do this to move forward in my life and heal. Now that I have forgiven I will continue my life in a positive way.

Once you have forgiven, you must realize that it is so and truly work to put the blame behind you. Only then can you move forward in your healing.

Figure 8.4 Forgiveness Exercise.

CHAPTER 9

THE MOLECULAR CHANNEL

Occasionally, my students in anatomy and physiology will explore how medications elicit their effects on the body. I will present a hypothetical situation whereby they are taking a medication. They know the medication is broken down and assimilated by the digestive system and subsequently travels through the bloodstream. The problem is how does the medication know where to go? What does it do when it gets there? How is this similar to or different from taking a vitamin?

Usually, after a bit of a struggle, we end up with the answers. The medication knows where to go because of cellular receptors. Cells contain proteins imbedded in their membranes that act as receptors. The medication works like the body's own hormones and neurotransmitters by fitting into these receptors, much like a key fits into a lock.

Vitamins work a bit differently. They do not mimic hormones or neurotransmitters. Vitamins are needed for many of the chemical reactions in the body. Vitamins, commonly called coenzymes, work to make these reactions happen.

What is remarkable about both medications and vitamins is that what they transfer to the body is essentially information. Both contain messages that are taken in by the cells and tissues of the body. A message can tell a cell to do many different things. The cell can increase or decrease a particular process. It can make more message-containing proteins or secrete a variety of substances. These cellular messages can have widespread effects on the body. They can promote healing or they can wreak havoc and cause harm to cells and tissues.

Medications and vitamins are not the only molecular information sources. Virtually anything that goes into your body can transfer molecular information. This includes minerals, herbal substances, and even food. It also includes alternative remedies such as essential oils.

Molecular information moves through the body by what we will call the molecular channel. The channel consists of a source of molecular information such as a medication, a pathway such as the bloodstream, and a receiver such as a cell. The sources of information we will explore are medications, vitamins, minerals, and herbs.

With the understanding that medications, vitamins, minerals, and herbs all transfer molecular information, some of the differences between alternative and mainstream treatments begin to dissolve. For example, the general thinking is that nutrients and medications work differently. Yes, they may have a different *effect,* but the underlying mechanism of information transfer is essentially the same.

Both nutrients and medications transfer information. Both have their place in healing. The difference lies in the *content* of the information.

Medications as Information Sources

Medications carry molecular information much like the body's own hormones and neurotransmitters. Medications are powerful information carriers—perhaps too powerful in some cases—because they produce so many unwanted side effects. Many people take medications unaware of the side effects, and often the side effects are treated with still more medication. Drug manufacturers' advertising downplays the side effects—ads show happy people enjoying the benefits of a medication with only a brief mention of the side effects. It is difficult to grasp the seriousness of the side effects when watching laughing, smiling people enjoying life.

Side effects are known as adverse drug reactions, or ADRs. The number of ADRs is astounding. A recent review of research examining ADRs determined that close to 2.2 million occur annually. If we combine the incidence of ADRs with medical errors, the chance of having a serious injury when entering the hospital is as high as 36 percent! A review conducted in 2003 determined that 19 percent of 400 patients experienced an ADR upon discharge from a highly specialized hospital.[1]

This does not take into account unreported events. Adding these would push the numbers much higher since only 5 percent to 20 percent of these events are actually reported. A study published in the prestigious *New England Journal of Medicine* showed that 25 percent of patients demonstrated side effects from the greater than 3.34 billion medications prescribed that year.[2] The study went on to state that the medications causing the highest number of side effects included NSAIDs (non-steroidal anti-inflammatories), calcium channel blockers, and selective serotonin reuptake inhibitors (SSRIs) such as paroxetine (Paxil) and setraline (Zoloft). A report by Reuters also suggested that over one million hospital admissions per year are the result of side effects.[3] In many cases, doctors have a difficult time determining whether a patient's symptoms are due to an illness or side effects.

All medications are toxic to a certain degree. If you ingest enough of virtually any medication, you will exhibit signs of toxicity to the point of death. The amount of medication taken is called the *dose*. If the dose is too small, there will be no response. If you increase the dose, eventually it will be high enough to cause a response. The response increases with higher amounts of medication until a therapeutic effect is reached. Toxic effects result from doses higher than the therapeutic dose.

Medication works best through a range of doses, from the minimum amount needed to produce an effect to the level that is toxic. Some medications require a "loading" dose to prime the system or to get the enough of the drug into the bloodstream so that smaller doses can follow. Using a loading dose helps to maintain a constant supply of the medication to the cells.

The appropriate dose of a particular medication is generally determined by the weight of the recipient. The practitioner usually starts with an average dose, then adjusts it according to the individual. The average dose is known as the median effective dose or ED_{50}. This dose will produce a therapeutic effect in 50 percent of a group of patients.

However, not all humans are the same. A much lower dose than average may cause a therapeutic effect in some people while a much higher dose causes this effect in others. In many cases the therapeutic effect is reported back verbally by the patient. This results in communication errors and can lead to higher doses than necessary.

We said earlier that all medications are toxic to some degree or another. An index of toxicity is known as the median lethal dose or LD_{50}. This index represents the dose that is lethal in 50 percent of patients. Both the ED_{50} and LD_{50} can be used to determine the therapeutic index:

$$Therapeutic\ Index = LD_{50}/ED_{50}$$

Some medications have a narrow therapeutic index. This means that the amount needed to produce a therapeutic effect is very close to the toxic amount. There is a greater likelihood for error in using a dose that is too high. Some examples of narrow therapeutic index drugs are illustrated in figure 9.1.

Medications may be manufactured to work like hormones or neurotransmitters, but there are some important differences. The natural process of hormone or neurotransmitter secretion is a finely tuned mechanism. The body is capable of secreting just the right amount of a substance to elicit just the right effect. There are numerous feedback mechanisms that are constantly adjusting the

Medications with a Narrow Therapeutic Index

Oral contraceptives

Antiepileptic drugs

Warfarin (a blood thinner)

Cisapride (for heartburn)

3-hydroxy-3-methylglutaryl coenzyme A reductase inhibitors
(commonly known as the statin drugs for lowering cholesterol)

Flouroquinolone (an antibiotic)

Tricyclic antidepressants

Figure 9.1 Medications with a narrow therapeutic index.

amount of hormone secreted. Medications generally overwhelm these regulatory mechanisms.

Medications tend to bombard the molecular channel with information. The information is not as finely adjusted as the natural information carriers. Medications can cause widespread effects because they may fit many receptors located throughout the body. It is difficult to finely tune dosages so they compare with the natural production and secretion of hormones.

A quote by neurophysiologist Candace Pert illustrates this concept:

"Avoid exogenous ligands (drugs) that perturb the psychosomatic network so much that they warp its smooth information flow, producing 'stuck' information circuits that prevent you from experiencing your full repertoire of potential experiences, and instead cultivate feedback loops that restore and maintain your natural bliss. Translation: To feel as good as possible all of the time, avoid doing drugs, legal or illegal. Question any chronic prescription: If you have to have it, make sure you are taking the lowest possible dose that does the job."[4]

Many side effects could be reduced if there were a way to more specifically adjust the dose of a drug. There is hope for this in a new branch of pharmacology called genetic-based pharmacology or pharmacoge-netics. The way an individual responds to a drug depends on their DNA, since DNA holds the instructions for producing enzymes that break down drugs in the body. In some people the instructions are slightly different, causing their DNA to produce variations of these enzymes. In these people a small dose of medication can have lethal effects.

Genetic testing will be capable of identifying those individuals who will benefit from a medication and those who can be harmed. Some people metabolize medications faster than others and need higher doses to achieve a therapeutic effect. Others metabolize medications more slowly, and medications given to them can cause a toxic effect.

The future is bright for genetic testing and pharmacology. It is interesting that the concept of an individually specific dose based on genetics is, in essence, an informational approach based on DNA.

Vitamins and Minerals as Information Sources

Vitamins and minerals (nutrients) work differently on the body from medications. Nutrients are commonly called natural substances because they are used in normal biochemical processes. Nutrients are contained in the foods we eat and are necessary for normal physi-ology. Vitamins generally function as coenzymes in the body. Coen-zymes make possible many of the biochemical reactions in the body.

For example, the body uses a simple carbohydrate called glucose for energy. The biochemical reactions that produce energy from glu-cose require the B vitamins riboflavin and niacin. In this way vitamins enable the processing of the foods we eat. Without vitamins the body could not metabolize carbohydrates, fats, and proteins.

The body does not make vitamins, so they must be ingested in the diet. Some vitamins are synthesized by the skin such as vitamin D or by intestinal bacteria (vitamin K). Vitamins come in two broad categories, water-soluble and fat-soluble. Water-soluble vitamins are absorbed and excreted within a short time of ingestion. They are not stored in body tissues. Fat-soluble vitamins are stored in the body along with fat. There is a greater danger of toxicity with fat-soluble vitamins.

Some vitamins, including C, E, and A, work as antioxidants that combine with free radicals to disable them. Free radicals are toxic molecules produced by chemical reactions in the body and can be harmful.

The body also needs minerals. The body needs seven minerals in moderate amounts, and a number of other minerals are needed in small or trace amounts. The seven minerals are phosphorus, calcium, potassium, sulfur, chlorine, sodium, and magnesium. Minerals are used to strengthen bone, produce cell membranes, and form proteins, hormones, and enzymes.

Since vitamins and minerals are part of the normal physiological processes in the body, they can be integrated into the molecular information flow better than drugs.

You can think of nutritional substances as working to support the normal biochemistry of the body in contrast to medications that either overwhelm or suppress it. Medications flood the molecular information channel much like a conquering army, whereas nutritional substances provide information much like a supply line. That is not to say that nutrients are perfectly safe as they exhibit toxic effects at a high dose level, just like drugs. However, their toxicity is much lower than that of drugs.

An article published in the *Journal of Orthomolecular Medicine* examined the number of deaths associated with nutrient overdose and found that the incidence was 0–1 per year. The article went on to state that in over 49,000 exposures to vitamins reported to poison control centers, there were only *"fourteen major adverse outcomes and no deaths."* The authors went on to state *"morbidity and mortality from pure vitamins are rare."* [5]

Herbal Supplements as Information Sources

Herbal supplements provide molecular information much like medications. In fact, many of today's medications were developed from herbs. The drug form is much more refined and potent than the actual herb.

Herbs have been used as medicinal substances for thousands of years. It may be that herbs are better suited as information sources because they have coevolved with humans.

Herbs can be categorized according to their effects on the human body. Adaptogens, such as ginseng and astragalus root, work to support normal physiological processes in the body. An adaptogen increases immunity, supports liver function, increases stamina, and decreases the effects of stress by supporting adrenal function. Antioxidants such as grape seed extract combine with free radicals to disable them. Carminatives have a calming effect on the gastrointestinal system and are used for irritable bowel syndrome, heartburn, indigestion, and infantile colic. Examples of carminatives include peppermint and ginger. Cholagogues such as dandelion and burdock root stimulate the production and flow of bile. Demulcents support the function of mucous membranes. Some demulcents include licorice root and marshmallow. Laxatives such as aloe vera increase the action of the colon.

The use of nutritional and herbal remedies continues to grow in the United States. Herbal remedies have always been more popular in Asia and Europe but the U.S. is catching up. Herbal remedies contain a lower dose of the active ingredient than medicines. They may also contain a variety of active ingredients. In some cases the combination of ingredients works together to support the desired effect on the body. There are many herbal substances with a variety of effects on human biochemistry. Many mechanisms of action are still unknown and are being discovered.

Herbs are generally safe, but there are some reports of adverse reactions. According to a report by the FDA, there were 184 deaths associated with herbal substances reported between 1993 and 1998. This works out to thirty-seven deaths per year. Most of these were attributed to weight-loss formulas that contained an herbal stimulant known as ephedra. [6]

Biologicals

A relatively new class of substances called biologicals offers tremendous potential in healing. Biologicals use the body's own immune system to fight diseases. Where nutritionals and herbal substances support physiological processes, biologicals actually participate more closely in the body's physiology. In terms of resonance, biologicals closely match the natural information sources of the body.

Biologicals consist of molecular substances produced by the body, including antibodies, interleukins, interferon, genetic material (gene therapy), vaccines, and colony-stimulating factors. All of these are called biological response modifiers (BRMs). Many of these substances are being developed for use in cancer treatment and are capable of targeting cancer cells directly or helping the immune system destroy the cells. Another group called nonspecific immunomodulating substances stimulate immune system function. These substances will cause the immune system to produce more antibodies and cytokines that are capable of attacking cancer cells.

Since biologicals closely match substances that the body already produces, there is hope that they will cause fewer and less severe side effects. At present, side effects do exist and can range from mild to severe. However, traditional chemotherapy also produces numerous side effects while it is less specific in targeting cancer cells.

One category of biologicals called monoclonal antibodies work by targeting the cancer cells. The body's B-lymphocytes (a type of white blood cell) naturally produce antibodies when activated by a pathogen such as a virus or bacteria. The antibodies then attack the pathogen and make it more recognizable for other cells to attack. Monoclonal antibodies work in much the same way. When injected into the body, the antibodies specifically target cancer cells so the immune system can work to eliminate them.

Vaccines work by introducing a disabled pathogen into the body so the immune system can respond by naturally producing antibodies against the pathogen. Cancer vaccines are being developed that contain a portion of a person's own cancer cells that have been disabled.

Injecting these back into the person stimulates the immune system to attack the cancer cells.

In gene therapy, genetic material is presented to the body by injecting viruses that contain the material. The viruses are disabled so they cannot cause a disease. One approach involves supplying missing genes to the DNA in cells. It is thought that DNA that contains missing genes tends to produce cancer cells. Another approach involves introducing genes that enable the immune system to better recognize and fight off the cancer cells.

Choosing a Molecular Information Source

All of the above substances can be used as molecular information sources. Medications are very powerful and produce effects quickly. They are also dangerous, as they tend to overwhelm the body's natural processes. Herbs are less powerful and less likely to produce side effects. They can be considered natural remedies because they coevolved with humans. They affect the body more slowly than drugs and may have a more symbiotic effect. Nutrients are the least potent as they are already a part of the normal biochemical processes of the body.

There is much hope for the future of biologicals. Since these substances already exist in the body, they are powerful sources of information. If the source of a genetic disease is the DNA itself, then why not repair it? In the future this may be possible.

Drugs, nutrients, and herbals can all be valuable information sources in a healing program. In choosing a molecular information source the type and severity of the pathological mechanism must be considered. The problem with modern medicine is that these sources are not seen as equal. There is a tendency toward the overuse of drugs. The reasons for this are political, educational, and even commercial. Unfortunately our society suffers the consequence of too many adverse drug reactions.

Generally, it appears that the power of a substance is directly proportional to the side effects produced. Medications and biologicals are more powerful than their natural alternatives, but they produce the most side effects. The nutrients and herbal substances are less powerful but produce fewer side effects. Which to choose depends upon the pathological process. Questions to be considered include:

- Is the process acute or chronic?
- How severe is the process?
- What are the accepted treatments?
- What are the side effects?

For acute problems, a more powerful information source may be needed. In terms of information flow, acute problems can be thought of as powerful streams of information occurring in a specific area of the body. For example, acute inflammation is a cellular response to injury. The cellular inflammation programs are activated and send strong streams of information to the injured area. The most effective interruption of this process would result from the use of a drug, but then side effects would need to be considered. Use of natural alternatives could be considered if the inflammation is not severe. Another approach could be to use a medication for a short time, then change to a natural alternative.

For chronic problems, you should consider the use of alternative remedies as long-term use produces fewer side effects. Alternative remedies typically take longer to work as they produce a less severe result. When at all possible, the treatment should progress from using sources of information that have a more powerful effect to those having a lesser effect.

If more powerful sources of information are used to control an acute process, then the subsequent healing process should be supported by less powerful sources of information. For example, an acute flare-up of inflammation may require a medication, but this could be supported with nutritional or herbal substances.

To illustrate the use of molecular information, let us take a look at a specific case. Jasmine came to my office with acute neck pain that began shortly after a rear-end vehicle collision. She described the pain as sharp and severe. She said the pain increased with movement and radiated to her right shoulder and arm region. She had trouble sleeping due to the pain, and could not get comfortable. My examination revealed signs of an acute inflammatory process occurring in her neck musculature.

In order to control her inflammation I had several choices. I could use a nutritional anti-inflammatory such as bioflavonoid, or I could use medications of various strengths ranging from over-the-counter ibuprofen to one of prescription strength, such as hydrocodone (I usually refer patients to a medical practitioner for prescriptions). All of these substances act as sources of information, with some being more dangerous than others. The prescription strength variety also contains a narcotic for pain control. If I used the prescription medication I could control the inflammation quicker but risk more serious side effects such as drowsiness, nausea, and liver damage. Over-the-counter ibuprofen is less powerful, with fewer side effects, and the bioflavonoid is even less powerful with almost no side effects.

When I examined the benefits and cost of all three substances, I decided to use the over-the-counter ibuprofen along with a nutritional substance (bioflavonoid) for three days, then discontinue the drug while continuing the bioflavonoid. In this way the benefits were maximized while the risks were reduced. Figure 9.2 presents some suggestions for using nutritional substances.

The most severe problems in the body, such as cancer, require a regimen of powerful information sources. Cancer cells create a large amount of entropy in the body. It takes a lot of information to overcome this process. Many of the latest cancer treatments include powerful chemotherapeutic drugs along with nutritional support. All of the information sources must be evaluated regarding how effective they are at healing versus how damaging they are to the body.

My advice for using molecular sources of information is to take your time and research what you are using. There are some simple suggestions of nutritional substances for various problems presented in figure 9.2. If you are considering taking nutritional substances along with medications it is important to check these out with your pharmacist. The increased use of nutrients and herbal substances has

Nutritional Substances for Healing

If you are experiencing any of the following diseases you may wish to explore the use of the following natural substances. This list is not a substitute for professional care but serves as a general guide. If you are interested in taking any of these substances you should work with your professional health care provider. Never reduce doses of medication without consulting the practitioner who prescribed them.

If you have high blood pressure you may consider taking:

- Vitamin E (400–800 i.u. daily)
- Carnitine (1000–3000 mg daily)
- Coenzyme Q10 (30–90 mg daily)
- Garlic (fresh or capsules)
- Dandelion
- Hawthorn

For controlling pain and inflammation:

- Bioflavonoid
- Digestive enzymes
- Cayenne pepper
- White Willow Bark
- Feverfew (for headaches)
- Ginger
- Tumeric
- Boswellia

Figure 9.2 Nutritional Substances for Healing (continued on next page).

resulted in an increased awareness of interactions with medications. Your pharmacist can be an important resource for identifying these.

There are a number of licensed practitioners who use nutrients and herbal substances to heal. I would advise anyone to seek help from one of these people who have advanced knowledge of these substances. Many times such substances can be used in conjunction with or even in place of medications.

Nutritional Substances for Healing (continued)

For joint damage and osteoarthritis use the above to help to reduce pain along with glucosamine sulfate (1500 mg daily). The glucosamine has been shown to reduce the degeneration of the joints.

For carpal tunnel syndrome use the above to help control pain and inflammation along with vitamin B6 (50–100 mg daily).

If you are having problems sleeping you may consider taking:

- Valerian root
- Melatonin
- Calcium (600 mg)
- Magnesium (300 mg)
- Kava root (for anxiety that prevents sleep)

For prostate problems such as benign prostatic hyperplasia:

- Zinc (10–15 mg daily)
- Selenium (200–400 mcg daily)
- Saw palmetto

For acid indigestion:

- Licorice root extract (deglycyrrizinated licorice)
- Slippery elm
- Marshmallow root
- Methylsulfonylmethane (MSM)

Figure 9.2 Nutritional Substances for Healing .

Molecular information is a powerful addition to a complete healing program. As presented in chapter two, molecular information works through upward causation to affect the body. Although molecular information is powerful, it is important to remember that the molecular information sources should be part of an overall healing program that includes the use of the other channels.

CHAPTER 10

THE ENERGY CHANNEL

Energy is everywhere. Every time we listen to beautiful music, enjoy the view of a spectacular landscape, or feel the hardness of wood we are receiving energy. Energy not only allows us to experience the world outside of our bodies but also can help us to heal.

When you listen to music, what you experience is your mind's interpretation of sound waves rippling through the air. The sound waves strike your eardrum and the vibrations are transferred to your inner ear. Your inner ear converts the mechanical energy to electrochemical energy in the form of nerve impulses. The nerve impulses enter your brain and your brain interprets them as music. The entire process is an example of energy converted to information.

All of your senses function this way. They gather information in the form of energy from the environment and convert it to electrochemical information for use by the nervous system. We take in enormous amounts of information in the form of energy every day. Our nervous systems then have to sort it out and put it into context.

Life, Energy, and Information

Life needs energy. Life was able to begin and evolve on this planet because it had an energy source, the sun. Much of the energy needed to support life comes from light, heat, and chemical molecules. Life is able to extract the information from energy and integrate it into its structure.

Energy in its essence is force. In physics a force is the capacity to invoke a change in something. There are four fundamental forces in nature: gravity, strong nuclear, weak nuclear, and electromagnetic forces. In healing we are most concerned with the electromagnetic force.

The electromagnetic force involves more than electricity and magnetism, as its name implies. Most of the science of chemistry involves the action of the electromagnetic force. In chemical reactions molecular bonds are broken and new ones formed. The electromagnetic force produces chemical bonds.

Much of what our senses take in comes from the electromagnetic force. The light we see, the sound we hear, the textures we feel are all examples of this force. It is responsible for giving hardness to a substance like a block of wood or softness to a pillow. It has also been used in healing for more than one hundred years.

Electrical Energy as Information

In the early 1900s, it was thought that delivering electrical energy to the body in the form of a shock was a good thing. Electromedicine was quite popular at this time and was considered a high-technology medicine. There was even a medical subspecialty with an organization entitled the American Electrotherapeutic Association that held annual meetings and conferences. It was around this time that inventor Nikola

Tesla had been experimenting with alternating current and high-frequency electrical energy. Tesla was famous for developing alternating current for the transmission of electricity over long distances.

Tesla also discovered that he could pass a large amount of electrical energy through the human body using high-frequency current. He described the human tissues as acting as condensers that could store electrical energy. He also knew that cells were electrical in nature. He knew they maintained an electrical gradient, a difference in voltage between the inside and outside of the cell. He thought that he could help to maintain or even improve on the cell's function by exposing the body to his high-voltage, high-frequency current, so he constructed *healing* devices called Tesla coils that produced this current, with the goals of restoring health and even curing cancer. Tesla's devices gained huge popularity inspiring other inventors to produce offshoots of his original device. Many of these devices can now be seen in museums. Tesla so believed in his theory that he exposed himself to the current daily.

All living cells exhibit a difference in voltage between the outside and inside of the cell. Cells typically have a negative potential inside the cell as compared to outside. This difference in potential is created by the passage of ions across the cell membrane. It is called the transmembrane potential. A high-voltage, high-frequency electromagnetic field appears to stimulate the cell and support the normal transmembrane potential. This potential is linked to important cellular processes such as the production of energy and normal cell metabolism. Diseased cells such as in cancer have been shown to have a decrease in transmembrane potential.

Tesla coils also produce ozone and negative ions, which can be beneficial to living tissue in small amounts. Negative ions act somewhat like an antibiotic and can destroy pathogens. They also boost the immune system. Ozone (ionized oxygen) has also been found to have health benefits in small amounts. Other effects include an increase in DNA and protein synthesis and a decrease in pain.

Using Very Small Currents to Heal

In contrast to high-voltage, high-frequency electricity, very small currents have been found to promote healing. Much of the work on small currents, known as microcurrents, was inspired by the work of Robert Becker, a medical doctor.

It was known for a long time that damaged tissue produces a current of injury, which was thought to be charged atoms (ions) leaking out of the tissue. The current of injury supposedly decreased as the tissue healed. Dr. Becker, an orthopedist and author of the book *The Body Electric*, thought this current was related to the regenerative properties of the tissue.[1] His idea inspired a series of experiments with frogs and salamanders designed to investigate whether currents could promote the regeneration of limbs.

Becker's ideas were not well received by the scientific community. His ideas about regeneration went against the accepted thinking that regeneration could not occur because once cells developed from their precursor cells (stem cells) they could not reverse this process. Differentiation was seen as a one-way street, at least in human cells. Once the cell differentiated, it could not develop in the other direction. Becker was intrigued, however, by the idea that it might be possible for cells to be stimulated to regenerate where regeneration was not supposed to happen. His first project was not met with enthusiasm. The professor who needed to approve his project even said:

> *I don't believe for one minute that it will work, but I think you should do it anyway. We need to encourage young researchers.*[2]

Becker's first project compared the regenerative properties of salamanders to frogs. Salamanders have the ability to regenerate limbs while frogs do not. He found that he could partially regenerate the limbs of frogs by changing the polarity of an amputated limb.

Becker showed that the current of injury had nothing to do with leaking ions from damaged tissue but was somehow related to the healing properties of tissue. He went on to study the effects of microcurrent on human tissue with great success. He was able to develop a device that accelerated healing in fractures that is used by orthopedic doctors. He was also able to retard the growth of cancer cells, using silver electrodes and a positive current.

What Becker found was a way to send healing information to the tissues of the body in the form of electromagnetic energy.

He states:

I postulated a primitive...information system...that...used semiconducting direct currents and that, either alone or in concert with the nerve impulse system, it regulated growth, healing, and perhaps other basic processes.[3]

Herbert Fröhlich, a researcher at the University of Liverpool, also investigated communication among cells. He proposed the existence of a cellular communication system that used vibrations and waves to synchronize protein synthesis.[4] He thought that when cellular molecules vibrated in unison they formed a kind of communication network.

The search for a cellular communication system was inspired by the lack of a complete explanation of how DNA and the cell carry on such enormous and complicated tasks. There are thousands of processes going on in a cell at any one moment and all occur in harmony. The mystery lies in what directs these processes to make them work so well. Like a large factory producing protein products, cells must have some sort of communication from management. Instructions must be sent throughout all levels of the organization in order to orchestrate the complex production lines, packaging, shipping, ordering raw materials, and so on. It was originally thought that DNA was all the management the cell needed.

We may think information flows in a top-down manner from president to vice president to manager to worker. However, there are also many feedback loops to consider as communication occurs in the other direction. This is where the DNA management falls short. The information flow from DNA occurs primarily in one direction—from DNA outward. Without feedback, DNA alone could not handle the complex network of feedback loops. Therefore, Becker and Fröhlich searched for another way for cells to communicate.

The work of Tesla, Becker, Fröhlich, and others provided the impetus for a variety of energy devices on the market today. Some of these are readily available to anyone; others need to be administered by a qualified practitioner. All can be considered sources of information in the form of energy. I will focus on just a few of the many devices available. These include microcurrent, magnets, interferential current, low-powered lasers.

Microcurrent

Microcurrent devices are closely associated with Becker's work on the healing currents of the body. These devices work by gently assisting the body's normal current with a very small therapeutic current. The cells of the body contain membranes that allow the passage of ions in and out of the cell. This is the transmembrane potential as described above. The application of small currents seems to support these potentials. Research has shown microcurrent increases cellular energy.[5]

Microcurrent seems to be especially beneficial in decreasing pain. A number of studies have shown that pain decreases and tissues heal faster when microcurrent is used, either alone or in conjunction with other treatments.

Chiropractors, physical therapists, and some medical doctors use microcurrent. There are larger stand-alone devices as well as smaller portable devices that can be taken home. The devices produce a very small current that is not felt by the patient. Electrodes are attached to the body so that the current passes through the area to be healed. The portable devices allow for frequent treatment sessions that can be done by the patient. As shown in figure 10.1, microcurrent is effective in treating a number of disorders.

Magnets

Magnets have been a source of healing information and controversy for many years. The use of magnets for healing extends back 2,000 years. Research regarding magnets and healing is scant in the United States, but there are hundreds of studies in Europe and Russia. One

---

Disorders Effectively Treated with Microcurrent

Arthritis

Generalized pain

Sprains and strains

Bone regeneration

Temporomandibular joint disorder

Trigger points

Circulatory disorders

Swelling

Wound healing

Musculoskeletal disorders

Figure 10.1 Disorders effectively treated with microcurrent.[6]

recent study published in the *British Medical Journal* suggests that magnetic bracelets are effective in reducing the pain from osteoarthritis.[6] Magnets seem to be most effective in promoting healing in musculoskeletal problems and in reducing chronic pain. Magnets are used in Japan to treat chronic fatigue syndrome. Some acupuncture treatments include the use of magnets over meridians.

One study examining the effectiveness of using magnets for knee pain found that 85 percent of those surveyed experienced at least a 50 percent reduction in pain.[7] Another looked at using magnets for menstrual pain and found that 90 percent of women using a certain brand of magnet still had a reduction in pain after one year. Nearly 50 percent of these women had a reduction in pain of at least 70 percent.[8]

There is some discrepancy in the research regarding which pole of the magnet to use for certain conditions, and there are some contraindications. Magnets should not be used during pregnancy, cancer, with a pacemaker, or near open wounds.[9]

Strong magnets of greater than 500 gauss are recommended for penetrating human tissue for healing. So far there have been no side

Disorders Effectively Treated with Magnets

Chronic pain	Inflammation	Nervous system problems
Fractures	Stress	Asthma
Bronchitis	Carpal tunnel	Arthritis
Depression	Swelling	Fibromyalgia
Circulatory problems	Strains/sprains	Post-polio

Figure 10.2 Disorders effectively treated with magnets.

effects reported with the use of magnets. Figure 10.2 illustrates a number of disorders that respond to magnets.

Just how magnets work is not known. Some theories suggest that magnets assist the normal electrical current of the body and promote healing of cells. Others have seen an increase in blood flow to an injured area. Recently, magnetic material called magnetite has been found in the human brain. Magnetite has been known to exist in animal brains and contributes to their ability to navigate. One way magnets may work is by interrupting the processing of pain signals in the brain.

Generally people use magnets by attaching them to the body over the painful area. Some studies recommend intermittent use and others continuous use. There are many magnets on the market used by a variety of alternative healthcare providers. If you are thinking of using magnets, the best advice I can give is to get in touch with a professional health-care practitioner who has experience using magnets.

Interferential Current

Interferential current (IFC) has been around since the 1950s and is a popular modality in physical therapy. It is used by medical doctors, physical therapists, and chiropractors to stimulate healing in nervous and musculoskeletal problems and has shown very good effectiveness in treating these conditions. IFC is approved by the FDA and is reimbursable by the majority of insurance carriers. IFC is a low level cur-

---

Disorders Effectively Treated with Inferential Current

Chronic pain	Swelling	Arthritis
Myofascial pain	Neuritis	Inflammation
Sprains/Strains	Fractures	

Figure 10.3 Disorders effectively treated with inferential current.

rent with variable frequency capable of penetrating body tissues to elicit healing. Figure 10.3 illustrates a number of disorders that have responded to IFC.

IFC should not be used when pregnant in treating cancer, open wounds, or infections; with pacemakers; or for deep vein thrombosis. IFC may stimulate the production of the body's own pain modulators such as endorphins and enkephalins, which help to decrease pain. IFC is safe with virtually no side effects.[10] A typical IFC session consists of attaching electrodes to the body across the area of pain. The session lasts around ten minutes and is painless. I have used IFC on myself for healing and I enjoy the soothing feeling of the current.

Light

Light is also a form of electromagnetic radiation. Humans need light for chemical reactions that produce vitamin D in the body. Also, light has long been known to promote healing. In the absence of light, many people suffer from a condition known as seasonal affective disorder (SAD). SAD causes mild depression during the darker winter months. People suffering from SAD find relief by sitting in front of a bright light source.

Other kinds of light that have healing properties include ultraviolet and infrared light. Ultraviolet light has been known for its antibacterial properties for many years. Infrared light and microwaves have been used for their ability to raise the temperature of body tissues to promote circulation and cellular activity.

In general, light with lower frequencies has more therapeutic properties than high-frequency light. High-frequency, low-wavelength light tends to destroy organic tissue. An example of this is the gamma radiation produced by linear accelerators in cancer treatment. The devices produce a precise beam of high-energy photons targeted at a specific area of cancerous tissue with the goal of destroying it.

Most light, especially the light we see, is composed of many frequencies. It wasn't until 1960 that a source of single frequency (coherent) light was produced. That year Theodore Maiman constructed a device that produced a red monochromatic light. The device was named after what it does: Light Amplification by Stimulated Emission of Radiation, or LASER for short.

The laser was initially seen as a potential weapon of science-fiction proportions. In the biomedical realm high-power lasers were seen as a source that could be focused to precisely destroy tissue such as cancerous tumors. Thus, research focused on high-power lasers. But what about the healing power of low-power lasers? Could low-power lasers facilitate healing?

Dr. Endre Mester was a Hungarian physician who was especially interested in developing a laser for medical use. He used a specially built red laser on rats that had tumors. When he exposed the tumor cells to his laser he found the tumor cells were not destroyed as he thought. The skin incisions he had made to insert the tumor cells had actually healed faster. This led to a series of experiments with the goal of stimulating faster healing in surgical incisions. His experiments were successful in speeding up the healing of incisions. It turns out that Mester's laser was not as powerful as he thought. It was a low-powered laser in contrast to the high-powered, tissue-destroying lasers.[11]

Mester's laser was the first to stimulate healing of living tissue. A number of experiments conducted since have shown that low-powered lasers of different wavelengths can promote healing of a variety of tissues including cartilage, bone, muscle, nerve, ligaments, and, of course, skin. The wavelength that promotes healing is between 600 and 1000 nanometers. The healing benefits include decreasing inflammation, stimulation of new cell growth and blood vessels, and speeding up the cellular repair process. Low-power lasers have even been shown to promote cell growth in healing resistant ulcers. [12]

Lasers may work on living tissue through the presence of certain light-absorbing molecules in the cells. Examples of these are porphyrins, cytochrome c, chromophores, and flavins. These molecules are located in the cell membrane and in an organelle that produces energy called the mitochondrion. It appears that these molecules can store the energy provided by the laser light and increase the production of adenosine triphosphate, a chemical that functions as an important energy source for cells. ATP is used for many cellular processes including DNA, RNA, and protein synthesis. Increasing the production of cellular ATP is like giving the cell more fuel to do its work. As a result, the cell increases its function and productivity.

Low-power laser light also affects the nervous system, specifically the nerves that carry pain impulses. Patients undergoing a treatment regimen of low-powered lasers report less pain. One mechanism that may account for the decrease in pain is that the light somehow causes decreased secretion of a hormone called *prostaglandin*. Prostaglandins modulate pain. Another is the regeneration of nerve cells. Nerve cells regenerate faster after laser treatments. Figure 10.4 illustrates some disorders that respond to laser therapy.

Disorders Effectively Treated with Low-level Laser Therapy

Carpal tunnel syndrome	Joint pain	Plantar fascitis
TMJ	Sprains/strains	Tendonitis
Trigger points	Fibromyalgia	Migraine headaches
Neuralgia	Swelling	Myofascial pain
Post-operative pain	Bursitis	Wound healing

Figure 10.4 Disorders effectively treated with low-level laser therapy.

Low-powered lasers could be used as a source of information as part of an overall healing program. There are virtually no side effects reported so far due to the low level of energy. Chiropractors, physical therapists, and medical doctors use laser therapy for the treatment of muscular pain. A treatment session consists of attaching a device containing a number of laser diodes to the area of pain. The treatment is painless and lasts a few minutes to one half hour.

Mechanical Energy

Besides a host of energy-producing devices, we cannot forget about mechanical energy administered by an experienced practitioner. Mechanical energy is another manifestation of the electromagnetic force. Examples include bodywork, chiropractic, and music therapy.

In bodywork, information is conveyed to the body in the form of touch. There is a lot of information in the administration of force by experienced bodyworkers. They must pay attention to such things as the location on the body, the depth of the therapy, and the duration. The body receives these forces to correct tissue imbalances and increase circulation.

There are many kinds of bodywork, too numerous to cover in this book. Some examples are massage therapy, Trager, craniosacral, trigger-point therapy, and muscle energy techniques.

Music also carries information in the form of the electromagnetic force. Sound consists of differences in air pressure that produces waves. The pressure waves result from molecules of air colliding with each other. When air molecules collide they exchange forces. Music is rich with information carried by the electromagnetic force.

Music therapy has been found to be beneficial in reducing stress, pain, and high blood pressure. It also promotes a generalized feeling of well-being. Music therapy has been found to successfully treat developmentally disabled individuals as a way to improve function. There is not one type of music that works for everyone. For example, classical music may soothe one person, but irritate another. To find out more about music therapy, contact a qualified music therapist. You can also check out the American Music Therapy Association.

Chiropractic has been around in the United States for more than 100 years. The primary treatment performed by chiropractors is spinal manipulation. Historically, spinal manipulation is much older than chiropractic, and there is evidence that it began more than 2,000 years ago. Manipulation is also described in the writings of Hippocrates (460–357 BC).[13]

The beginning of chiropractic practice in the United States is attributed to the efforts of Daniel David Palmer, known as D. D. Palmer. Palmer had devised a method of healing that incorporated magnetic healing. His approach integrated mind, body, and spirit, which he called the "triune" approach. He set up an infirmary in Davenport, Iowa, which was very successful, and he gained many referrals from satisfied patients. He was never content with his success and continued to seek out new methods of healing.

One day in September of 1895 he began a conversation with Harvey Lillard, a janitor in his building. Lillard was deaf and communicated by using sign language. Lillard told him that seventeen years earlier he became deaf when he bent over and felt a "pop" in his back. Palmer examined him and discovered a lump on his back. Palmer deduced that if he could reduce the lump it might help Lillard's condition.

Palmer delivered a forceful thrust to Lillard's spine and after a number of treatments, Lillard could hear a ticking watch. Palmer then began to examine the spines of all of his patients, reducing what he thought were misalignments. He met with great success and the profession of chiropractic was born. He subsequently set up a school in Davenport that bears his name. Today chiropractors are classified as primary care providers and represent the largest organized group of alternative medicine providers.

The central treatment given by chiropractors consists of an adjustment. Delivering a mechanical force to a joint, most commonly a joint in the spine, makes the adjustment. The idea is that the joint can become stuck or fixated as well as out of position, in what is called a *subluxation*. The adjustment helps to correct these problems. Chiropractors also use a number of the modalities described above such as microcurrent, interferential current, and lasers.

Chiropractors believe that there is an intimate link between the spinal joints and the nervous system. Correcting a problematic spinal joint helps the nervous system function better.

In terms of information we can describe an improperly functioning joint as having a greater degree of disorganization or entropy than one that is functioning well. The adjustment provides information in the form of mechanical force to reduce entropy and restore normal functioning. The reduction in entropy is experienced in the body, and the body functions better.

We must pay attention to the concept of resonance when using energy. We need to send just the right amount of healing information to the body. Too much causes damage, while too little is not enough to promote healing.

When I first began to see a chiropractor many years ago, I was fortunate to have chosen a very skilled practitioner. I always felt better after the treatments and looked forward to going. One day, during a treatment session, he told me that he was going on vacation and would not be seeing patients the following week. It was important that I continue my treatment so he arranged for another chiropractor to treat me that week. I went to my appointment looking forward to getting my adjustment and once again feeling better. The substitute chiropractor had a good personality and was confident in administering the treatment. He performed exactly the same adjustments as my chiropractor. I remember him moving my body in exactly the same way and pushing on the same areas of my spine. The only difference was that he used a significantly greater amount of force.

I felt okay when I left the office, but not nearly as good as I usually did after a treatment. The next day I woke up feeling as if I'd been hit by a truck! My whole body ached. This lasted for about two days. I was really looking forward to the return of my regular chiropractor.

The point is that both performed exactly the same treatment with very different results. Perhaps my body was bombarded with too much information by the substitute chiropractor. Mechanical force, like all healing modalities, is an information source. Attention must be paid to resonance. Skilled practitioners know this.

Information in the form of energy can be used in virtually any healing program. Energy, like molecular information, works through upward causation and can be a valuable addition to overall healing. Pay particular attention to resonance when using energy devices or seeing practitioners. In many cases, lower doses work better than higher doses with devices. With practitioners, experience is the key to resonance.

CHAPTER 11

USING THE KEYS

We have covered a lot of ground so far. We have learned how the body uses information to maintain itself and how we can tap into many sources of healing information by using channels. We learned about resonance and using feedback to fine-tune the flow of information. It is now time to put all of these principles into one program, a program you can use to heal.

This chapter is devoted to presenting all of the information in this book in the form of a powerful system of healing you can easily use. You will begin by reviewing the keys from chapter three. Then you will use the informational healing flowchart that organizes all of the keys. You can follow along step by step, recording your progress and adjusting your program along the way.

Reviewing the Keys

To summarize, the seven keys of informational healing are:

Key #1: Use healing intention first.

Key #2: Healing information flows from a source to a receiver through a channel.

Key #3: Use all four informational healing channels.

Key #4: The information source and receiver must be matched as closely as possible.

Key #5: Your consciousness automatically seeks healing information.

Key #6: Create a hierarchy of information sources.

Key #7: Fine-tune information flow with feedback.

A flowchart is presented in figure 11.1 that organizes the keys into a system you can use to put together your own healing program. Begin with key number one by writing your healing intention as described in chapter six. Use the exercise in figure 6.1. It is extremely important to declare your intention to heal, as this defines your purpose and provides motivation and direction for your healing.

Next you will complete a self-evaluation. This will give you much-needed feedback as informational systems change according to feedback. It is best to describe your problem in terms of how you feel emotionally and physically, as well as what you are thinking about your problem. To evaluate yourself emotionally, you need to write about your feelings regarding your problem. This may take some self-reflection. For example, when I was experiencing my problem I had feelings of denial, anger, and sadness. These feelings receded as I progressed until they were as diminished as my physical symptoms.

To evaluate your state of mind you need to write about your thoughts regarding your problem. It is important to identify whether you are internally or externally motivated (see chapters seven and eight) as well as any negative thoughts about your illness. For example, let's say that by completing this exercise you discovered that on a deep level you had thoughts about living a life of illness because

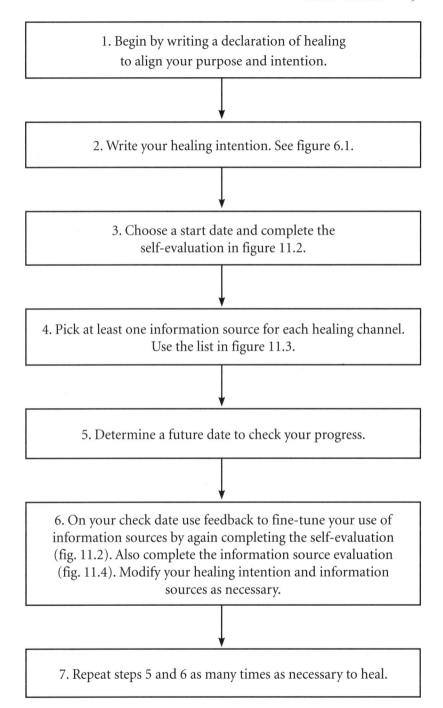

Figure 11.1 The Informational Healing Flowchart.

The Self-Evaluation

Evaluate your condition by writing about how you feel with regard to the following:

Emotional

How do you feel about your condition on an emotional level?

_____

_____

_____

_____

Mind

What do you think about your condition?

_____

_____

_____

_____

Physical

How do you feel physically? Specifically address pain and discomfort by describing the area of your body that is in pain, the quality of the pain (sharp, dull, burning, aching), and its intensity on a scale from 1–10, with 1 representing no pain and 10 representing debilitating pain. Put an X on the line between 1 and 10 to indicate your level of pain.

_____

_____

_____

_____

_____

Area of Pain: _____ Rating ⊦ – – – – – – – – –10
Area of Pain: _____ Rating ⊦ – – – – – – – – –10
Area of Pain: _____ Rating ⊦ – – – – – – – – –10

Figure 11.2 The Self-Evaluation.

you deserved it. You would need to engage these thoughts and explore them in order to fully heal (see chapter eight). Use the self-evaluation sheet in figure 11.2 to do this.

Evaluating yourself on a physical level will probably be the easiest. Here you will write about how you feel physically. You will address your pain and discomfort. There is an area for writing a general statement about your pain followed by an area that addresses specific locations of pain in your body. Here you can address the quality of your pain such as aching, burning, sharp, dull, or even numbing, as well as the intensity, by using the pain scale. There is room for three locations but feel free to use additional paper to expand if you need to. You can rate your pain on a scale of one to ten by putting an "X" on the line between the numbers. One usually represents no pain and ten represents excruciating pain.

Once you have finished the self-evaluation you can select information sources corresponding to each information channel. It is best to use at least one source of information for each channel. You can use more if you wish, but you need to be careful not to overload your system. A list is provided on the following pages in figure 11.3. I realize that not all modalities are listed and I apologize if I have left out a modality you are using. There are hundreds of healing modalities that can be used as information sources and it is difficult to categorize each one, as each requires a good understanding of how it works. Therefore, the list will serve as a guideline for you to choose modalities. You may wish to speak with practitioners about whatever modality you are using in order to get more detailed information as to how it works. Some modalities are used individually and others will be used in conjunction with a practitioner.

You will also see that some modalities are listed in more than one category. This is because some actually provide information using more than one channel. For example, Ayurvedic medicine is listed under nonlocal and molecular information sources. Ayurvedic medicine works on the nonlocal level, with its categorization of personalities as well as on the molecular level, with its herbal remedies.

Information Sources List

Use the following list to categorize the information sources you are using.

Nonlocal

Intention	Reflexology
Prayer	Aura Analysis
Meditation	Ayurvedic Medicine
Homeopathy	Acupressure
Acupuncture	Angelic Healing
Chi Gong	Bach Flower Remedies
Yoga	Bioenergetic Synchronization Technique
Network Chiropractic	Biodynamic Psychology
Bioenergetics	Body Mapping
Chakra Breathing	Chinese Medicine
Crystal Healing	Enneagram Analysis
Meridian Therapy	Macrobiotics
Naturopathy	Pranic Healing
Psycho-neuro-integration	Reiki
Shamanic Healing	Spiritual Psychology
Sufi Healing	Therapeutic Touch
Vibrational Healing	

Mind-Body

Imagery	Creative Visualization
Hypnosis	Integrative Therapy
Positive Thinking	Receptive Imagery
Body-Mind Centering	Silva Mind Control

Figure 11.3 Information Sources List (continued on next page).

Information Sources List (continued)

Molecular

Nutrients	Aromatherapy
Herbals	Diets
Medication	Naturopathy
Essential Oils	Orthomolecular Therapy
Ayurvedic Medicine	

Energy

Cold Laser	Rolfing
Magnets	Alexander Technique
Ultrasound	Trager
Electrical Muscle Stimulation	Craniosacral
Microcurrent	Color Therapy
Surgery	Music
Chiropractic	Heat
Physical Therapy	Ice
Massage Therapy	Radionics

Note: Some modalities are listed in more than one category if they use more than one information source.

Figure 11.3 continued.

Next, you must choose a time to again measure your progress. This will depend on the severity of your problem. In my practice, I generally check in with patients every visit and formally evaluate them about once a month. You will need to give your healing program some time to work, but I would not recommend waiting longer than one month to evaluate. Once your chosen time period passes, you will review what you have written about how you were feeling when you began, and then complete another self-evaluation. You will also evaluate each of the information sources to determine how useful you think they are. There is a worksheet for this also in figure 11.4. An

Information Source Evaluation

List the information sources you will use for each channel. Use the list on pages 154–155 as a guide. Use the effectiveness scale to rate each one when you complete your evaluation.

Nonlocal

1:_____

        1 2 3 4 5

2:_____

        1 2 3 4 5

3:_____

        1 2 3 4 5

Mind-Body

1:_____

        1 2 3 4 5

2:_____

        1 2 3 4 5

3:_____

        1 2 3 4 5

Molecular

1:_____

        1 2 3 4 5

2:_____

        1 2 3 4 5

3:_____

        1 2 3 4 5

Energy

1:_____

        1 2 3 4 5

2:_____

        1 2 3 4 5

3:_____

        1 2 3 4 5

Figure 11.4 Information Source Evaluation.

easy way to do this is to rate each modality on a scale from one to five; one being the lowest level of effectiveness and five being the highest. This will help you to add, subtract, or modify modalities from your program. For example, you may work with your physician to decrease the amount of medication you are taking, or you may wish to rewrite your healing intention.

You will then set another date to evaluate and repeat the entire process as many times as necessary. Remember this is a process and it will require time to complete. It is important to exercise patience. Healing is a non-linear process and exacerbations or setbacks are common and even expected. You need to stay the course and give it more time. During this process you will be adding healing information using all of the channels as you go along, and using feedback to change in a positive way.

My Healing

When I reflected on my own healing from the heart disorder I described in chapter one, I realized it incorporated all of the concepts of informational healing. I did not know this at the time and there was much trial and error along the way.

One of the important things I discovered was that my healing needed to occur on several levels. Before the illness I was on a path to destruction. I was not in touch with myself, but living on a superficial plane of existence. My purpose was wrong and I was in denial about my limits, my health, and what I truly needed. I worked too long and too hard at my job and put my health too low on my list of priorities. My purpose was to be successful at all costs. The crisis was a wake-up call for me to change.

My healing began on a molecular level with taking medications to suppress symptoms. These medications did not actually help me heal on that level, but they did allow me to function well enough to work on other aspects of healing. I continued to heal with the inclusion of a number of nutritional substances over a period of several years. I began with a multivitamin. This was not in the usual pill form but was a powder that was mixed with juice for better assimilation. I supplemented this with a variety of nutrients that improve heart function, such as coenzyme Q10, beta carotene, selenium, vitamins E and C, and omega-3 fatty acids. I also improved my diet. I gave up caffeine and ate more balanced meals, with much less processed food and more vegetables.

I used mind-body techniques, the same as those presented in this book. These were awkward at first and took a long time to master. I used tapes, music, and even recorded myself reading imagery exercises. I did not experience an instantaneous improvement or remission of the problem, but I gradually experienced a deep knowing that I would eventually heal.

The mind-body exercises also brought to light certain unhealthy thought processes buried deep in my subconscious. As these surfaced I was forced to deal with them to stay on my purpose to heal. Denial of these thoughts would contradict that purpose. As a result I experienced personal growth as well as healing. To heal I needed to have a healthy mind.

I first learned about the importance of healing intention when attending professional school to become a chiropractor. By this time I had few symptoms, but I still had problems on occasion and was still taking medications. I decided to use healing intention along with meditation on a regular basis. I wrote my intentions down and reflected on them frequently. My consciousness could then accept nonlocal healing information. The entire healing process did not happen overnight. From the time of my initial diagnosis to when I felt I was healed took almost ten years. My cardiologist conducted a number of tests on my heart and said there was no evidence of my original problem, confirming my healing.

Since I began this journey into healing I have witnessed thousands of people experience healing at various levels. People who were most successful used techniques much like those presented here. I believe those who were not as successful could have experienced better results if they had used this system of healing.

If you follow the system you will heal too. Once you use the keys to heal, information will flow to you as it did to my patients and me. You must be patient and consistent in your efforts—since healing, in many cases, does not occur overnight. Many small steps over time can add up to big results. I would like to personally wish you the best in your own healing journey.

CHAPTER 12

HEALING STORIES

The following is a collection of true healing stories from people I have met while researching this work. Some are personal friends, others coworkers and patients. They represent a sample of the thousands of people I have treated and known. Every time I work with someone I learn something more about healing and I am grateful to each one for what they have given me. All of these stories share common elements of using information to heal. Each represents a piece of the informational healing system. Each person was able to somehow tap into one or more sources of healing information to reduce entropy in their bodies. What is remarkable is they did so without using mainstream medicine.

Tracy and the Nonlocal Channel

Tracy is a vibrant and active person who holds down a full-time job and has an eight-year-old son who also keeps her busy. Her life changed when she began to suffer excruciating pain from a herniated disc. Many of the daily activities we all take for granted produced severe pain. She sought help for her problem from what was considered to be the best care in the area, a large medical spine center. The center has a comprehensive approach to back problems and includes a variety of medical specialists, physical therapists, and even a chiropractor.

On her first visit she was in so much pain that she could not even lie down on the examining table. After the examination and an MRI, the doctor told her the unwelcome news that she needed spinal surgery, saying, "You are going to be in a body cast for three months!" And even then there were no guarantees.

Concerned about her prognosis, Tracy wanted to take some time to think about the surgical option and subsequent period of disability. She did not want to rush to make such an important decision but she felt she did not have much choice. One day soon after the grim news, a coworker took her aside and said, "Hey, how would you like to get healed?" Tracy was amazed and didn't think this was possible. The coworker told her about the pastor of a local church who could heal the sick. Skeptical, but willing to try anything, Tracy decided to go to meet this healer. She was still in pain at the time and her friend had to drive.

The church was located in an older section of town (ironically, a large modern hospital was just down the street). The building was reminiscent of an old Catholic school with a built-in church, circa the 1940s. A makeshift sign on the lawn displayed the times of the services. One entered the building by passing through a grand entrance with a pair of oversized wooden doors under a large concrete cross.

Tracy describes meeting the pastor as follows:

Just by looking at him I could tell he seemed very warm and very honest, and he just started talking about healing from the Bible and quoting the Bible, and he really knew the book itself. There were a lot of people sitting there and I remember I couldn't even sit on the chairs they had. The whole time I stood, and when all was said and done, about an hour of preaching ... he asked if

*there was anyone who needed healing. And right away I came for-
ward and he put his hands on me and the other people began to
speak in tongues and also put their hands on me. The pastor said,
"When I take my hands off, you will no longer have any pain."
And I wanted to believe it and I thought there was something
going on with everyone speaking in tongues, which I have never
experienced before. I kind of felt something, but I didn't totally
believe it. So they stopped praying and told me to do something
I couldn't normally do. So I bent forward and back. I thought,
wow, the pain was gone! After the service I was even able so sit on
a wooden chair without pain.*

Tracy experienced immediate relief from her pain. The pastor told
her that she might need further healing if her pain came back and
to call if this happened. One day soon after, Tracy's pain returned
while at work. She immediately called the pastor and he told her to
go somewhere private where they could pray together. She took the
phone into a vacant conference room where she continued speaking
with the pastor. He told her to put her hand on her leg where she was
having pain, and they prayed together. Again her pain disappeared.

Sometime later the pain returned and Tracy again contacted the
pastor, this time through his web site. The pastor encouraged those
who needed healing to contact the web site and put their names on
a list. During the Thursday night service he would hold up the list
of those who needed healing from the web site so the congregation
could pray for them. Tracy's pain began on a Tuesday and continued
through to Thursday. On Friday the pain was gone. Tracy was anxious
to tell the pastor when she returned for the Friday service she frequently attended. She entered and he pointed to her and said, "I know
you are feeling better because we prayed for you last night."

By now, Tracy was a firm believer. The pastor told her she needed
to continue to pray and read the Bible as she could also lose her healing. She believed so much in her healing that she took her son Alex
to the church. Alex was a longtime asthma sufferer and was taking
a number of medications. Anytime he was sick from a cold or virus

he suffered a major asthma attack. The pastor told her she needed to trust in her belief that her son would be healed—so much so that she needed to take him off of all medications! Tracy was frightened at the prospect of this, as she had seen how severe his attacks had been. She tried taking him off of the medications a couple of times only to cave in out of fear and take him to back to the doctor, who naturally put him back on the drugs.

The pastor again told her to trust in her belief and take her son off of all of the medications. Tracy recalls:

> *So I did and I believe when people say God speaks to your heart. I just believed when Alex coughed … I heard God say to my heart—he is healed. He coughed one more time and I heard again—he is healed. And then I believed. I am the kind of person where God would have to put a note in my mailbox. I needed proof. Ever since I felt that God spoke to me, I knew. So when Alex came down with anything I took him to the asthma and allergy clinic and had him tested. This happened twice and both times they said he just had a virus. Before his healing he would always have a severe asthma attack whenever he had a cold or flu. Now Alex believes he is healed and says, "Mom, I don't have asthma anymore."*

Tracy's case is a great example of the power of the mysterious nonlocal channel. This channel can send healing information to anyone, at any time at any location. It is not dependent on time as information is transferred instantaneously. The nonlocal channel began to open the instant Tracy decided to go to the church. Her intention to heal was present despite her skepticism. Her intention became stronger when she met the pastor. She experienced a deep knowing that he could help.

The pastor brought up an important point about healing. He said that one had to continue to believe and that healing could be lost. His method for supporting healing was through Bible study and prayer. If you lost your way in your belief, then you could risk losing your healing. This process of supporting healing with belief constitutes a continuous supply of information. If the body is moving toward greater disorganization and information is needed to keep it from doing so, then why not supply information with intention and belief?

In Tracy and Alex's cases the information flow was so powerful that nothing else was necessary to support healing. No medications, physical therapy, or surgery were needed.

Lisa and the Mind-Body Channel

Lisa lived a healthy life. As an alternative health care practitioner she knew the benefits of exercising, eating well, and keeping stress under control. A former professional dancer, Lisa continued her involvement in dance by teaching ballet, and she loved ballroom dancing. Besides the usual aches and pains resulting from an active lifestyle, Lisa had no reason to see a doctor. That was until she began to notice some gynecological problems that she thought warranted a medical opinion. She decided to see her gynecologist for a checkup.

The doctor performed a routine pelvic examination and mammogram. Lisa was concerned about the pelvic problems. She did not realize that soon they would be her least concern. The mammogram results showed the presence of a tumor. A subsequent biopsy confirmed the grim diagnosis of cancer.

Lisa needed a few days to process the impact of having cancer. She decided to get a second opinion. A second doctor agreed that she had breast cancer. Like many cancer victims, Lisa had a difficult time accepting her diagnosis. When I asked her how she felt when she found out she had cancer, she said that she felt numb.

Her doctor recommended she see a surgeon who wanted to schedule her for breast surgery, followed by a regimen of radiation therapy. Faced with these prospects, Lisa decided to do something that many of us would find difficult if not impossible to do. She decided to take a path that few have traveled. Lisa decided to exclusively use alternative medicine to try to heal from her cancer.

Her decision to take an alternative route was inspired by her work in holistic healing and her negative experiences with the medical approach. Even though her sister was a nurse and her brother-in-law a doctor, she did not have enough trust in medicine to accept her doctor's recommendations. Some of her family members were vehemently opposed to her rejection of medical treatment. They firmly believed in the medical system and tried to persuade and even control her. Ironically, her brother-in-law took a neutral stance. Lisa was left to embark on her path alone, with only the help of her alternative practitioners.

She began by reading a number of books on using alternative medicine to heal from cancer. She also sought the help of a naturopath, a homeopath, a Reiki master, a hypnotherapist, and a prayer group. Her treatment regimen included herbals, nutrients, homeopathic remedies, bodywork, and energy healing. She underwent a painful course of treatment using an escharotic salve. The salve burrows deep into the skin and destroys the cancer, leaving a gaping wound that scars over. The process generally takes from a few weeks to months.

When I asked her about her treatment she said that the most important things she used were daily imagery sessions and the unconditional support she received from her alternative practitioners and prayer group. She engaged in frequent imagery sessions. She used tapes to help her visualize ridding her body of cancer and seeing herself healed. She included many positive images and statements in these sessions. She felt that they not only helped her body combat the disease but also kept her in a positive state of mind.

Her prayer group also helped to support her emotionally and spiritually. She attended weekly sessions where she and others shared their experiences with their problems. These sessions were not only helpful in providing support but also helpful in getting at the emotional roots of the disease. They helped to bring certain thoughts and feelings to the surface so that they could be dealt with.

About nine months after beginning her intensive regimen of alternative medicine, her homeopath and naturopath both agreed, without each other knowing, that she was cancer free. Despite her resistance to medical treatment she gave in to her mother's pressure to have a lumpectomy and second biopsy. She insisted that her doctor perform it. Her doctor, who practiced complementary medicine, could not believe the results of the biopsy taken at the same site. He called her and said *"there's been a miracle...there is no evidence of cancer!"* A second doctor confirmed the results of the biopsy. Lisa was cancer free.

Lisa credits her healing to her alternative practitioners and her strong purpose in her life. She said that the reason she became a massage therapist was for this moment, so that she could deal with her cancer in this way. Her work had enabled her to see the power of alternative healing so that she could follow her path despite the opposition of her family.

Lisa continues to get checked periodically by her alternative practitioners and now, seven years later, she has remained cancer free. Lisa continues her work in helping others to heal and is now working on becoming a teacher of yoga.

My interview with Lisa affirmed the importance of using the mind-body channel to heal. Her intention and belief in her treatment, as well as her daily use of mind-body techniques, allowed her mind to become a powerful source of healing information. Although she used a variety of treatments, she credits the mind-body work for keeping her motivated and in a positive state so that she could complete her healing.

William and the Energy Channel

A long-time back pain sufferer, William experienced several episodes of pain so severe he had to lay on the floor with his legs elevated to get any relief. Conversations with friends discouraged his pursuing the conventional medical route.

The stories I heard from older guys with chronic back pain scared me away from traditional healing methods as I was not interested in either drugs or surgery.

William thought these painful episodes were unusual as he was a healthy college instructor in his thirties. He did not work a physical job nor did anything that he considered detrimental to his back.

A friend recommended he see a chiropractor so William consulted the local yellow pages and found one nearby. After a few treatments he began to feel somewhat better—however, the pain continued. This went on for five years. There were pain-free periods with occasional bouts of severe pain. William became discouraged as he was faced with living with this problem for possibly the rest of his life.

An avid basketball player, William would participate in pickup games at the local YMCA. This was his primary form of exercise and was a nice break from teaching. During one game a friend recommended he try another chiropractor. William knew him as the chiropractor also played basketball. He made the change and began to see this new practitioner.

I immediately felt better. It seemed like they both used similar techniques, but the second doctor, first of all, sympathetically listened to my descriptions of the symptoms and activities that led up to the injuries ... I liked the guy and I trusted him.

William is now in his fifties. He gave up basketball about ten years ago, mostly because his knees began to bother him. In place of basketball, William attends regular exercise classes and says:

My back is in far better shape than it was twenty years ago.

A few years ago William's problems took a new direction. He began to develop severe neck and shoulder pain.

My family MD suggested it was the beginnings of arthritis and prescribed muscle relaxants. They made me drowsy and were ineffective anyway.

William again went to the chiropractor who successfully treated his back pain, but this time the results were not as good.

The stretching exercises prescribed by my friend, the chiropractor, helped somewhat, but minor pain would come and go, often related to stress and long hours of grading student papers.

At a stress seminar William spoke with a massage therapist who thought his problem might be related to muscular tension. He tried a massage and it proved to be very effective and eliminated most of the pain. William learned that his body reacted to stress by making his muscles tight and painful.

Since I am a regular meditator, you would think I would have known that, but … so soon old, so late smart. Therefore, I have added massage to my routine of walking and stretching, I have very little shoulder pain. Since then I have added a moderate weight-lifting routine and my upper body feels better for that, too.

William's use of the energy channel, combined with his intention to heal, produced a powerful flow of healing information.

William's experience illustrates several important points about informational healing and using the energy channel. First, William's intention to heal was an important factor. It may seem obvious that pain would motivate someone to heal, but there is an important difference between merely managing pain and healing. I have seen many people who take medications to reduce pain and are in dire need of healing. These people often respond to even small degrees of healing. William actually wanted to heal from his problem, not just cover up the symptoms.

Second, William experienced resonance with the second chiropractor. Even though both administered the same treatment, the second was more effective. William trusted this fellow and connected with him. This practitioner listened to his problem and also had the intention to heal. Patient and practitioner are more effective when they resonate (see chapter four) as healing information flows more readily. Resonance can be as simple as having trust in your practitioner.

William also used more than one modality to heal. Besides the chiropractic treatments, he also exercised and meditated to reduce stress. We learned in chapter three that information should come from more than one source. In William's case, information flowed through the energy channel and the nonlocal channel. William also could have used the molecular channel by taking some nutrients or herbal substances, and the mind-body channel by incorporating a technique such as imagery into his meditation sessions.

Lastly, William used feedback. His healing only progressed so far with the first chiropractor. He realized this and sought out someone else. When the second chiropractor could not help his neck and shoulder pain he added a massage therapist to his healing regimen.

William had no knowledge of informational healing, but intuitively used a number of the keys. His extensive use of the energy channel was instrumental in helping him heal. By doing so, he experienced a greater degree of healing than when he followed the traditional route of care.

Steven and the Molecular Channel

Steven is a cancer survivor. His experience with cancer began not with his own health, but with his wife's. About thirty years ago she contracted a serious form of cancer at the age of forty. In order to get the best care available, she followed a treatment plan that relied exclusively on the advice of her physicians. The treatment included the usual surgery, radiation, and chemotherapy. Steven was forced to stand by her and watch her deteriorate. The entire process took about three years before she passed away. In my interview with him he recalled that time:

> Those were a horrendous three years, and I'm sure her dying had a negative experience on our two young children.

Steven began to see the traditional medical approach to cancer in a negative light. Witnessing a close friend and neighbor succumb to cancer reinforced his negative view. Both followed the traditional medical treatment model. Both had hopes of remission followed by acceptance of mutilation and severe pain before death.

Then about five years ago Steven received the dreaded news that he also had cancer. A routine medical checkup had uncovered prostate cancer. The checkup included a blood test called the PSA (prostate specific antigen). The results indicated a higher than normal PSA level that increased the possibility of cancer. Faced with the prospect of going through what his wife and friends did, he decided to take a different approach to his care. He began by visiting a naturopathic physician in order to get a picture of his overall health. The naturopath performed some tests that showed evidence of cancer. A follow-up with his medical physician included a rectal exam and a biopsy. Both were positive for cancer.

Steven was faced with the same decisions his wife and friends had struggled with. Should he too have surgery, radiation, and chemotherapy? Would he eventually succumb to the disease in the same way as the others?

He commented about these issues:

In a way this was a positive happening because it was now my life, not my advice, which would serve as an example for others if I survived and prospered. I didn't want to die painfully under doctors' care when I could do that on my own, so I chose to seek alternative solutions.

Steven decided to exclusively follow an alternative medicine treatment plan. By doing so he felt he had more control over his health.

I thought I was living a healthy life, having given up smoking and alcohol years ago, but I learned that I still wasn't living pure. I decided to treat myself nutritionally and emotionally.

His treatment consisted of a regimen of organic foods, juices, nutrients, exercise, and colonics. He consumes mainly fresh, raw foods purchased from a local co-op as well as delivered from an organic farm. Here is a sample of his nutritional program:

A naturopath recommended the following for lunch every day: Sprouted buckwheat and sprouted beans (to form a whole vegetarian protein), kale, parsley, cilantro, onion, garlic, avocado, lemon, miso (fermented raw beans), and seaweed. These raw foods are put into a blender and ground up to make a cool green soup for lunch.

Here's another recommendation that I follow. Every night I soak nuts and seeds (walnuts, almonds, sesame, pumpkin, and sunflower) for eight hours so that the live enzymes can be released by morning. They are put into a blender with raw fermented cabbage (which is high in flora), garlic, buckwheat and bean sprouts, bee pollen, and dried herbs such as turmeric, ginger, rosemary, and fennel.

He also gets regular exercise, weekly bodywork from a massage therapist, and visits a Reiki practitioner once a month. Steven admits to getting discouraged once in a while and credits his partner for providing support. She also lost a spouse to cancer, and together they maintain their nutritional regimen.

Steven continues to get his prostate checked twice a year and continues to see a naturopath for a cancer screening. At this point, five years after his diagnosis, his PSA levels have lowered to within a normal range and his rectal exams show a slightly enlarged but soft prostate. During a follow-up interview he said that he knew of two other friends who contracted prostate cancer in the last five years. Both followed traditional regimens of care; both are now gone.

Steven's remarkable story is a great example of using a variety of information sources to help him heal. I give him a lot of credit for following his own path to healing. Many of us would be fearful to take such a path that is so different from the mainstream medical approach to treating such a potentially devastating disease.

There is a big difference in these two approaches that I hope you will realize. The medical approach to treating prostate cancer essentially consists of various forms of surgeries to remove the prostate followed by radiation and chemotherapy in order to destroy the remaining cancer cells. The survival rates are very good if the tumor is confined to the prostate. The question is whether this approach actually produces healing. In other words, if someone engages in an unhealthy lifestyle, does removal of a diseased organ constitute healing?

Surgery, radiation and chemotherapy are powerful information sources. They all function by destroying cells and tissue. Although this approach can be very beneficial in destroying the cancerous cells, the patient must also consider that he must heal from the treatment.

If we examine Steven's case with regard to informational healing we first see that he did not believe in the traditional medical approach. He had a strong purpose and intention to heal, but had little faith in surgery, radiation, and strong medications. Belief in a treatment is an important part of healing. Belief strengthens healing intention and helps to increase the flow of healing information through the mind-body channel.

Steven has made ample use of the molecular channel. All of the organic foods, nutrients, and cleansing (so that nutrients can be absorbed) provide a good source of molecular information to his body. In addition to his cancer remission, Steven now enjoys a healthier lifestyle.

Steven's belief in a creator helps nonlocal healing information flow from a higher source. He also has regular Reiki treatments. Reiki masters are excellent sources of nonlocal information. They act as pathways for the flow of nonlocal information directly from the information field.

Steven's regular visits to a massage therapist and chiropractor represent his use of the energy channel. The mechanical energy provided by a skilled practitioner can also be a powerful source of healing information.

Steven's treatment encompasses many of the keys of informational healing. He uses all of the information channels, gets feedback through regular checkups, and has a great intention to heal.

Each of the above stories provides valuable insights into the underlying mechanism of healing. In each case we see strong purpose and intention. We also see the use of information sources and the idea that healing is a process that must be supported by information. Each person experienced entropy in the form of disease. The underlying cause could have been faulty genetic information, lifestyle choices, or a mechanical breakdown of body systems. Whatever the cause, each person needed to find a way to reduce the entropy and move the body in a direction of organization. Information is the only thing that reduces entropy.

The informational healing process must be supported. As the pastor told Tracy, you can lose your healing if you lose your support. If the entropy has progressed to an advanced point such as in cancer, then a great amount of information will be needed to support the body.

I hope these cases will inspire you to use the informational healing system in your own healing. I know they have all contributed to my inspiration and continue to do so.

CHAPTER 13

THE FUTURE OF
INFORMATIONAL HEALING

Can mainstream and alternative medicine, two disparate systems with large philosophical differences, ever be fully united? Will patients someday experience a system that encompasses all of the healing channels? It is my belief that such a system is possible and more likely to evolve with a universal theory of healing at its core. This theory will integrate new ideas from our fundamental understanding of the universe. It will define healing in a way that is compatible with all systems of healing.

Our present healthcare system presents a disjointed approach to healing. In many cases therapies are directed toward reducing pain or controlling symptoms with little regard for actual healing. This seems to be the case more with chronic illnesses such as arthritis and heart disease. However, there are signs that this is beginning to change. The tide may be turning, as there is an increasing demand for alternative therapies. The roots of this change did not come from the medical establishment but from you and me, the consumers.

For years many of us were aware of alternative therapies and many of us used them to help us heal. There seemed to be somewhat of an underground movement toward the use of these treatments. The movement occurred without the medical establishment taking notice. That was until David Eisenberg, MD, a researcher at Harvard medical school, published a study on the use of alternative medicine that shocked the medical establishment. The study was published in the prestigious *New England Journal of Medicine* in 1993.[1] What was shocking about the results was that one in three Americans used some form of alternative treatment. The number of visits to alternative practitioners was so high that it exceeded the number of visits to medical doctors! This amounted to some thirteen billion dollars spent on alternative medicine yearly. The underground revolution was exposed.

Our federal government also took a large step when in 1991 Congress appropriated funding for the formation of the Office of Alternative Medicine to operate within the National Institute of Health. The organization had humble beginnings with a budget of about two million dollars, as compared to the billions spent on medical research, but it eventually grew into a formidable organization now known as the National Center for Complementary and Alternative Medicine (NCCAM), with an annual budget of about 120 million dollars.

The movement toward acceptance of alternative medicine evolved into what is now called *integrative medicine*. NCCAM defines integrative medicine as mainstream medicine combined with alternative therapies supported by scientific research. The growth of integrative medicine is evident with an increasing number of clinics and hospitals offering alternative treatments.

Many medical schools now offer some form of coursework in alternative medicine, including the prestigious Harvard, Johns Hopkins and Yale medical schools. According to a NCCAM report, more than half of the 125 medical schools in the United States now offer some form of education in alternative medicine.[2] This has occurred as a result of public demand for these services, which appears to continue to grow. A recent report examining the use of alternative therapies in the United States found that about 62 percent of all Americans have used some form of alternative therapy in a twelve-month period.[3] The most-used therapy was prayer for healing. Approximately 43 percent of people still used alternative therapies when prayer was omitted. The revolution was not only immense, but has grown to even larger proportions.

Signs of the demand for alternative therapies are everywhere. Turn on your television and there are commercials touting the benefits of vitamins and herbal remedies. An increasing number of newspaper and magazine articles discussing alternative treatments compete for our attention. The number of alternative medicine providers continues to grow. Even your local pharmacy has shelves containing alternative remedies.

The tide is indeed changing, but this change is occurring slowly within the medical establishment. The changes regarding the acceptance of alternative medicine are just beginning to trickle down to the grassroots level. I have been involved in this revolution from the beginning. I have seen some changes, but there is still a long way to go. From my perspective as a single practitioner working in a mid-sized midwestern city, I still experience resistance and animosity about providing alternative treatments. I see some large institutions including some alternative therapies but these are generally under the tight jurisdiction of the medical establishment. For example, one particular institution in the area hired a chiropractor as part of a team of providers including medical doctors, surgeons, and physical therapists. Patients must first go through the medical and physical therapies before they can see the chiropractor.

In one of my interviews with alternative practitioners, Lori, a massage therapist, related the story of one of her clients. The client was a man who fell off a ladder while cleaning his gutters. He fractured several vertebrae in his spine, shattering one completely. He subsequently was treated by a number of doctors as well as received extensive physical therapy. Although his fractured spine mended as most fractures do, he was left with debilitating pain and was released from care in this state.

One of this man's friends recommended he see a massage therapist, which led him to Lori. He began weekly treatments and in about a year's time his pain was brought down to a very low level and his function increased dramatically. He also decreased his use of pain medications and was able to perform many of the activities he had been unable to do he first began the massage treatments.

The point is that this man was released from the medical system without so much as a mention of any nonmedical alternatives. It was as if what was provided medically was the only treatment available. When that did not help, he was released to deal with his pain by taking medication. I have heard this kind of story many times. Often patients take the initiative to seek out my care, not because their medical doctors referred them but because they were unsatisfied with their care and decided to try something else as a last resort. Many of the practitioners I know have similar stories.

The alternative medicine side of the equation is not without fault either. Many alternative providers also contribute to the divide between the systems. Some do not refer to medical doctors for help in treating diseases that could benefit from medical care. Others are at all-out war with modern medicine. I have been to meetings and seminars in which everything from vaccines to surgery to pain medications were touted as damaging and dangerous to one's health. It was as if the millions of patients who benefited from these treatments were not considered.

Bridging the Systems

There is still a long way to go in getting both sides to work together. The problem as I see it is the lack of a common ground. One side describes healing in terms of scientific studies focusing on such topics as statistics, biochemistry, and surgery. The other describes healing in terms of energy, life force, chi, and individual clinical cases. Which side is correct? In my opinion they both are. Both sides contain truth in their principles and beliefs. All that is needed is a bridge to unite them so that they can communicate and work together.

The bridge is information. If healing is truly seen as an exchange of information then both sides have a common ground on which to stand together. All practitioners can work with the various channels in order to provide a more complete system of healing. Seemingly incompatible modalities such as chi gong and pharmacology will have a common ground. Chi gong, for example, works by manipulating vital energy. This energy in essence is information transferred using the nonlocal channel.

We have seen that medication, too, contains healing information that is transferred using the molecular channel. If more channels are used to provide information, perhaps less medication would be necessary. The more channels used, the less of each may be needed as sources of information.

Practitioners who understand informational healing can more easily communicate with each other, since they understand all healing modalities as manifestations of the same underlying process. Healing as information exchange should be taught in both mainstream medical *and* alternative medicine schools. For example, specialties may emerge in which practitioners learn to use a variety of modalities associated with one information channel. There would be those who only used nonlocal healing or those who only used the energy channel and so on. This informational approach to healing could even be made available through the present system.

Our present medical system has a long way to go to adopt such an approach, but it is not completely out of the question. Once there is a common ground from which to unify all approaches to healing there is at least a chance to move forward in a united way. It is my hope that someday we will all work together to develop healing systems based on information flow.

I believe that in the future we will hear a conversation between a medical doctor and alternative healer that uses terms such as medications, chi, surgery, and herbs. What is different about this conversation from the ones we hear at present is that both practitioners will actually *understand each other*. All of the elements of healing will be seen as information transfer through channels, and all will be valued parts of a healing program. The systems will be fully united to provide the best both have to offer.

As science moves forward toward a better understanding of matter and energy in terms of information, healing will follow. There are already signs that this is coming.

NOTES

Chapter 1: Day of the Cadavers
1. Schrödinger, 1967.

Chapter 2: Information Structures and Channels
1. László, 2004.
2. Akimov, et al., 1996.
3. Sheldrake, 2006.
4. Goswami, 2004.

Chapter 4: Making Healing Relationships Resonate
1. Cherry, 2003.

Chapter 5: The Mysterious Nonlocal Channel

1. Browne, 2004.
2. Dossey, 1997.
3. Peat, 1997.
4. Schmidt, 1970.
5. Schmidt, 1971.
6. Jahn and Dunne, 1987.
7. Nelson, et al.
8. Ibid.
9. Crawford, 2003.
10. Nash, 1984.
11. Grad, et al., 1961.
12. Braud and Schlitz, 1991.
13. Jahn et al., 1997.

Chapter 6: Using the Nonlocal Channel

1. Benson, 1975.
2. Orme-Johnson, 2001.
3. Dillbeck, et al., 1981.
4. Mearns, 2005.

Chapter 7: The Mind-Body Channel

1. Edelman and Tononi, 2000.
2. Putnam, 1987.
3. Dembrowski and Gurin, 1993.
4. Goodkin, 1986.
5. Schleifer, et al., 1983.
6. United States Dept. of Health, Education and Welfare. 1974.
7. Karasek, et al, 1982.
8. Bergrugge, L. M. 1982. Bruhn, et al., 1974. Karasek, et al.' 1988. Schnall, et al., 1992 (3), 1990.
9. Idler and Kasl, 1991.

10. Rossi, 1986.
11. Ibid.

Chapter 9: The Molecular Channel

1. Null, et al, 2005.
2. Alastair, et al., 1998.
3. Zuger, 1999.
4. Pert, 2003.
5. Rosenblum, 2005.
6. Hirshon, 2006.

Chapter 10: The Energy Channel

1. Becker, 1985.
2. Becker, Ibid p 71.
3. Becker, Ibid p 257.
4. Fröhlich, 1968.
5. Chen, et al, 1998.
6. Harlow, et al, 2004.
7. Eccles and Price, 2003.
8. Ibid.
9. Null, 2005.
10. Fourie, et al., 1992. Hurley, et al, 2001. Johnson, et al., 1999, 2001. Zizic, 1995.
11. Mester, et al., 1985.
12. Marovino, 2004.
13. American Chiropractic Association, 2005.

Chapter 13: The Future of Informational Healing

1. Eisenberg, et al., 1993.
2. National Center for Complimentary and Alternative Medicine. 2001.
3. Barnes, et al., 2004.

REFERENCES

Akimov, A. E., and G. I. Shipov. *Torsion Fields and their Experimental Manifestations*. Proceedings of International Conference: New Ideas in Natural Science, 1996. URL: http://www.eskimo.com/~billb/freenrg/tors/tors.html.

American Chiropractic Association. Retrieved on 3/11/05 at: http://www.amerchiro.org/media/whatis/history_chiro.shtml.

Barnes, P. M., E. Powell-Griner, K. McFann, R. L. Nahin. Complementary and alternative medicine use among adults: United States 2002. Adv. Data. 2004 May 27;(343):1–19.

Becker, R. O. *The Body Electric.* 1985. New York: William Morrow & Co.

Benson, H. *The Relaxation Response.* 1975. New York: William Morrow & Co.

Bergrugge, L. M. 1982. "Work satisfaction and physical health." *J. Community Health* 7:262–283.

Braud, W. G., and M. J. Schlitz. (1991). "Consciousness interactions with remote biological systems: Anomalous intentionality effects." *Subtle Energies: An Interdisciplinary Journal of Energetic and Informational Interactions.* 2, 1–46.

Browne, M. W. "Signal travels farther and faster than light." Retrieved on 11/11/04 at: http://www.cebaf.gov/news/internet/1997/spooky .html.

Bruhn, J. G., A. Paredes, C. A. Adsett, and S. Wolf. 1974. "Psychological predictors of sudden death in MI." *J. Psychosom.* Res. 18:187–191.

Chen, L., J. Tang, P. F. White, et al. "The effect of location of transcutaneous electrical nerve stimulation on postoperative opioid analgesic requirement; Accupoint versus nonaccupoint stimulation." *Anesth Analg* 1998; 87:1129–34.

Cherry, N. J. 2003. "Human intelligence: The brain, an electromagnetic system synchronised by the Schumann Resonance signal." *Medical Hypotheses* 60 (60):843–4.

Crawford., C, et al. "Alterations in Random Event Measures Associated with a Healing Practice." *Journal of Alternative and Complementary Medicine.* 2003, 9:345–353.

Dembrowski, Ted in Goleman, D., and J. Gurin, eds. *Mind Body Medicine.* 1993. New York: Consumer Reports Books, p. 69.

Dillbeck, M., G. Landrith, and D. Orme-Johnson. "The Transcendental Meditation program and crime rate change in a sample of forty-eight cities." *Journal of Crime and Justice*, 1981, 4: 25–45.

Dossey, L. 1997. "The Forces of Healing: Reflections on Energy, Consciousness, and the Beef Stroganoff Principle." Retrieved at: http://www.twm.co.nz/dossey1.html.

Eccles, N. K., and D. Price. "A survey to determine the effectiveness of *LegCare* on swollen and painful legs." www.magnopulse.com, 2003.

———. "A survey to determine the long-term effects of *LadyCare* static magnets on dysmenorrhoea (period pain)." www.magnopulse.com, 2003.

Edelman, G. M., and G. Tononi. *A Universe of Consciousness.* 2000. New York: Basic Books.

Eisenberg, D. M., R. C. Kessler, C. Foster, F. E. Norlock, D. R. Calkins, and T. L. Delbanco. "Unconventional medicine in the United States. Prevalence, costs, and patterns of use." *New England Journal of Medicine.* 1993 Jan 28;328(4):246–52.

Fourie, et al. "Stimulation of bone healing in new fractures of the tibial shaft using interferential currents." *Physiotherapy Research International.* 1992; 2(4):255–268.

Frohlich, H. (1968). "Long range coherence and energy storage in biological systems." *International Journal of Quantum Chemistry,* 2, pp. 641–649.

Goodkin, Karl in Wood, C. "Cancer: the mind matters—influence of cancer patients' attitudes." *Psychology Today,* Nov. 1986.

Goswami, Amit. *The Quantum Doctor.* 2004. Charlottesville, VA: Hampton Roads Publishing, p. 98.

Grad, B., et. al. "An unorthodox method of treatment on wound healing in mice." *International Journal of Parapsychology,* 1961: v3:5–24.

Harlow, T., C. Greaves, A. White, L. Brown, A. Hart, and E. Ernst (2004) "Randomised controlled trial of magnetic bracelets for relieving pain of osteoarthritis of the hip and knee." *British Medical Journal,* 329(7480):1450–4.

Hirshon, J. M. 2006. Mortality from Herbs. Retrieved on 1/12/05 from: http://www.emedicine.com/EMERG/topic449.htm

Hurley, et. al. "Interferential therapy electrode placement technique in acute low back pain: a preliminary investigation." *Arch Phys Med Rehabilitation* 2001; 82:485–93.

Idler, E. L., and S. Kasl. 1991. "Health perceptions and survival: do global evaluations of health status really predict mortality?" *Journal of Gerontology.* 46:S55–S65.

Jahn, R., B. Dunn, and R. Nelson. "Engineering anomalies research." *Journal of Scientific Exploration* 1987: 1:21–50.

Jahn R., et al. "Correlations of random binary sequences with pre-stated operator intention: A review of a 12-year program." *Journal of Scientific Exploration* 1997; 11:345–367.

Johnson, et al. "A single-blind placebo-controlled investigation into the analgesic effects of interferential currents on experimentally induced ischemic pain in healthy subjects." *Clinical Physiol & Func Im.* 2002; 187–96.

Johnson, et al. "A double-blind placebo-controlled investigation into the analgesic effects of interferential current (IFC) and transcutaneous electrical nerve stimulation (TENS) on cold induced pain in healthy subjects." *Physiotherapy Theory and Practice.* 1999;15:217–233.

Karasek, R. A., T. G. Theorell, J. Schwartz, C. Pieper, and L. Alfredsson. 1982. "Job, psychosocial factors and coronary heart disease." *Adv. Cardiol.* 29:62–67.

Karasek, R. A., T. Theorell, J. E. Schwartz, et al. 1988. "Job characteristics in relation to the prevalence of myocardial infarction in the U.S. Health Examination Survey (HES) and the Health and Nutrition Examination Survey (HANES)." *American Journal of Public Health* 78(8): 910–918.

László, E. *Science and the Akashic Field.* 2004. Rochester, NY: Inner Traditions, 50.

Marovino, T. "Cold Lasers in Pain Management." *Practical Pain Management:* Sept/Oct 2004.

Mearns, J. 2005. The Social Learning Theory of Julian Rotter. Retrieved on 11/20/04 from: http://psych.fullerton.edu/jmearns/rotter.htm.

Mester E., A. F. Mester, and A. Mester. "Lasers." *Surg Med*:1985:5:31–39.

Nash, Carroll B. "Test of psychokinetic control of bacterial mutation." *Journal of the American Society for Psychical Research,* 1984, 78(2), 145–152.

National Center for Complementary and Alternative Medicine. 2001. Report: Can Alternative Medicine Be Integrated into Mainstream Care? Retrieved on 6/15/06 from: http://nccam.nih.gov/news/past-meetings/012301/#4

Nelson, R. D., B. J. Dunne, and R. G. Jahn. *An REG Experiment With Large Database Capability, III: Operator Related Anomalies* (Technical Note PEAR 84003. Princeton Engineering Anomalies Research). Princeton, NJ.

Null, G. Biomagnetic Healing. Retrieved on 3/15/05 from: http://www.garynull.com/Documents/magnets.htm.

Null, G., C. Dean, M. Feldman, D. Rasio, and D. Smith. Death by Medicine, Part 1. Retrieved on 2/23/05 at: http://creativehealth.netfirms.com/death_by_medicine.shtml

Orme-Johnson, D. 2001. Summary of Scientific Research on The TRANSCENDENTAL MEDITATION and TM-SIDHI® Programs. Retrieved on 12/12/04 from: http://www.tm.org/research/summary.html.

Peat, F. D. 1997. An Interview with David Bohm. Retrieved on 3/2/05 from: http://www.fdavidpeat.com/interviews/bohm.htm.

Pert, C. B. *Molecules of Emotion*. 2003. New York: Scribner, p. 322.

Putnam, F. "Psychoneuroimmunology." *Noetic Sciences*, 1987; 4:4

Rosenblum, M. "Vitamin Toxicity." Retrieved on 2/25/05 from: http://www.educationplanet.com/search/cache?url=http://www.emedicine.com%2Femerg%2Ftopic638.htm

Rossi, E. L. *The Psychobiology of Mind-Body Healing.* 1986. New York: W. W. Norton & Company, 16.

Schleifer, S. J., S. E. Keller, M. Camerino, J. C. Thornton, and M. Stein. 1983. "Suppression of lymphocyte stimulation following bereavement." *Journal of the American Medical Assn.* 250:374-377.

Schmidt, H. "Quantum-Mechanical Random-Number Generator." *Journal of Applied Physics* 41, 1970, 462–468.

Schmidt, H. "Mental Influence on Random Events." *New Scientist and Science Journal,* June 24, 1971, 757–768.

Schnall, P. L., P. A. Landsbergis, C. F. Pieper, J. Schwartz, D. Dietz, W. Gerin, Y. Schlussel, K. Warren, and T. G. Pickering. 1992. "The impact of anticipation of job loss on worksite blood pressure." *American Journal of Industrial Medicine* 21:417–32.

Schnall, P. L., P. A. Landsbergis, J. E. Schwartz, K. Warren, and T. G. Pickering. 1992. "The relationship between job strain, ambulatory blood pressure and hypertension." Presented at the Ninth International Symposium on Epidemiology in Occupational Health, Cincinnati, OH.

Schnall, P. L., C. Pieper, J. E. Schwartz, R. A. Karasek, Y. Schlussel, R. B. Devereux, A. Ganau, M. Alderman, K. Warren, and T. G. Pickering. 1990. "The relationship between 'job strain,' workplace diastolic blood pressure, and left ventricular mass index: Results of a case-control study." *JAMA* 263:1929–35. Also, letter to the editor. *JAMA* 1992;267:1209.

Schnall, P. L., J. E. Schwartz, P. A. Landsbergis, K. Warren, and T. G. Pickering. 1992. "The relationship between job strain, alcohol and ambulatory blood pressure." *Hypertension* 19:488–94.

Schrödinger, E. *What is Life?* 1967. Cambridge, UK: Cambridge University Press, 71.

Sheldrake, Rupert. "Morphic Fields and Morphic Resonance, An Introduction." Retrieved on 1-21-06 from: http://www.sheldrake.org/papers/Morphic/morphic_intro.html).

United States Dept. of Health, Education and Welfare. 1974. *Work in America; Report of a Special Task Force to the Secretary of Health, Education and Welfare.* Cambridge, MA: MIT Press.

Wood, Alastair J. J. , et al. "Making Medicines Safer—The Need for an Independent Drug Safety Board," *New England Journal of Medicine* Vol. 339, No. 25 (December 17, 1998), 1851–1854.

Zizic, T. M. "Treatment of Osteoarthritis of the Knee with pulsed Electrical Stimulation." *Journal of Rhematology* 1995;22:1757–61.

Zuger, A. "Fever Pitch: Getting Doctors to Prescribe Is Big Business." *New York Times,* 1/11/99, pp. A1, A13.

GLOSSARY

Acetylcholine: A neurotransmitter secreted primarily by the parasympathetic nervous system.

Adaptogens: A class of herbal substances that help the body to "adapt" to stimuli such as stress.

ADH: Antidiuretic Hormone. A hormone secreted by the posterior pituitary gland that causes fluid retention.

ATP (adenosine triphosphate): An important energy-containing molecule in human physiology. ATP carries energy by virtue of its high-energy phosphate bond.

Basophil: A type of white blood cell containing large granules. Basophils are important in mediating inflammation and can release histamine and heparin. Histamine is a vasodilator that works to bring more blood to an area while heparin is a clotting inhibitor.

Bell's Theorem: A theorem proposed by J. S. Bell that stated the results of the Einstein, Podolski, and Rosen thought experiment could not be understood in terms of locality. According to the theorem, quantum action occurs nonlocally.

Bioflavonoids: A class of nutritional substances that have anti-inflammatory effects.

Biologicals: A class of substances that closely match substances in the human body. Examples of biologicals include antibodies, genetic material, cytokines, proteins, and vaccines. Biologicals are regulated by the FDA.

Biological response modifiers: A category of biological substances sometimes called biological agents that target specific cells to elicit a response.

Biomolecules: Carbon-containing molecules found in living systems.

Bohm's Theory: Also known as Bohm's Theory of Implicate Order indicates that there is a deeper connection between everything in the universe. David Bohm thought that there may be a deeper reality or interconnectedness that explains nonlocal quantum events.

Calcium channel blockers: A class of drugs that work to inhibit calcium channels in cells. Common calcium channel blockers include verapamil, bepridil, felodipine, and nimodipine. They work to reduce the workload on the heart.

Carminatives: A class of herbal substances that stimulate the digestive tract. Examples include: chamomile, ginger, fennel, and peppermint.

Carpal tunnel syndrome: Degenerative condition known as a peripheral neuropathy involving the median nerve. Causes pain, numbness, and tingling in the hand and fingers.

Cholegogues: A class of herbs that work to stimulate the production and flow of bile. Examples include: dandelion, burdock, artichoke, black root, barberry, and wild yam.

Chromophores: Substances that absorb electromagnetic energy in the form of light.

Circadian rhythms: Natural cycles of arousal and sleep.

Coenzyme: An organic substance that combines with a protein to form an active enzyme. Many vitamins work as coenzymes.

Colony-stimulating factors: A series of hormone-like substances that promote growth of blood cells in bone marrow.

Current of injury: Very small electrical currents (microcurrents) that are emitted from injured tissue.

Cytochrome c: A protein that can transfer electrons in an energy system in the cell known as the electron transport chain.

Cytokines: A series of substances secreted by immune system cells that work to activate white blood cells and attack pathogens.

Demulcents: A class of herbals that act as a protective barrier on membranes. Demulcents are typically used in the digestive or respiratory tract and have a soothing effect. They include: flaxseed, marshmallow, slippery elm, corn silk, and comfrey.

Electromagnetic: One of the four fundamental forces in nature. This force is carried by the photon.

Endorphins: A class of pain-modulating chemicals functioning as neurotransmitters or hormones. Endorphins work to decrease chronic pain.

Enkephalins: A class of pain-modulating chemicals functioning as neurotransmitters and hormones. Enkephalins work to decrease acute pain.

Entropy: A measure of the decrease in heat of a system. Also, the measure of disorder of a system.

Enzymes: Molecules that work to facilitate a chemical reaction by decreasing the activation energy of the reaction.

Epinephrine: A neurostransmitter or hormone that is secreted by the sympathetic nervous system. Important in eliciting the fight-or-flight response.

Free radicals: Reactive molecules that contain an unpaired electron. Free radicals cause cellular damage by taking electrons from molecules located in body tissues.

General Adaptation Syndrome: First described by Hans Selye in the 1920s, the General Adaptation Syndrome, or GAS, is a three-stage reaction to a stressful stimulus. The three stages are the alarm, resistance, and exhaustion stages.

Interferon: A class of immune system proteins that is capable of attacking pathogens such as cancer cells and stimulating other immune system cells. Interferons belong to a group of proteins called cytokines and are also known as biological response modifiers.

Interleukins: A class of immune system proteins that modify immune system responses. Interleukins belong to a group of proteins called cytokines and are also known as biological response modifiers.

LASER: Acronym for light amplified by stimulated emission of radiation. A Laser can produce light at a specific wavelength with no phase variations known as coherent light.

Manipulation: The art of providing mechanical force to move the tissues of the body. One of the most popular methods known as Chiropractic manipulation moves the joints of the body by the use of high-velocity, low-amplitude thrusts.

Mantra: A word or syllable used in the practice of meditation to assist in concentration.

Metaverse: According to László, the metaverse is the mother universe from which our present universe developed.

Microcurrent: A very small current in the microampere range.

Microwaves: Electromagnetic waves with a wavelength between .001 and .3 meters.

Multimodal healing: Using more than one healing process or modality.

Myofascial pain: Pain occurring in the muscles and associated fascial tissue.

Neuralgia: Pain originating in the nerves.

Neurodermatitis: A skin disease producing scaly, itchy patches of skin.

Neuroendocrine: A term used to describe the nervous and endocrine systems. Since the systems are so intimately linked the term is used in describing processes common to both systems.

Neuropeptides: Protein molecules that function as either neurotransmitters or hormones.

Neurotransmitter: A substance secreted by cells of the nervous system (neurons) for communication with other nervous system cells.

Non-steroid: A class of non-lipid soluble hormones.

Norepinephrine: A protein that acts as both a hormone and neurotransmitter. Norepinephrine is important in mediating the sympathetic nervous system (fight-or-flight) response.

NSAID: An acronym for non-steroidal anti-inflammatory drugs.

Percipient: An extremely sensitive person who may be capable of experiencing extrasensory phenomenon. Used in ESP experiments.

Photolysis: A process in which chemical bonds are broken by light.

Placebo: An inert substance.

Porhyrins: Molecules that are ring-shaped and function in the blood and respiratory systems.

Probability: The measure of the likelihood of the occurrence of an event.

Progressive muscle relaxation: A technique whereby groups of muscles are contracted and relaxed with the goal of reducing tension.

Psychoneuroimmunology: A branch of psychology that studies mind-body healing.

Quantum vacuum fluctuations: Also known as zero-point energy, the production of particle-antiparticle pairs in the vacuum of space.

Quarks: A subatomic building block of matter. Quarks come in six types known as flavors: up, down, strange, top, bottom, and charm.

Reiki: Developed by Mikao Usui in Japan, Reiki is a system of healing using the universal life force energy. The energy is transferred from the healer to a patient.

Relativity: Theory discovered by Albert Einstein that states the laws of physics are the same for any uniformly moving frame of reference.

RNA: Ribonucleic acid. RNA is important in transferring information from DNA outward to the cell and other cells in the body.

Self-efficacy: A person's belief that they will succeed at a task.

Shaman: A medicine man or witchdoctor who obtains power from the spiritual world.

Singularity: A region of space-time of infinite density.

Somatoemotional release: A muscle-release technique based on the premise that muscular restrictions harbor emotional problems.

Standard model: In physics, the model used to describe the fundamental constituents of matter and their interactions.

Steroid: A class of lipid-soluble hormones.

String Theory: A theory in physics that describes the fundamental unit of all matter and energy as tiny, one-dimensional vibrating strings.

Sympathetic nervous system: A division of the autonomic nervous system that can elicit the fight-or-flight response.

Transmembrane potential: Difference in electrical potential (voltage) between the inside and outside of a cell.

Tricyclic antidepressants: A class of antidepressant medications that affect neurotransmitter function in the brain. Examples include: imipramine, nortriptyline, and amitryptiline.

Trigger points: Painful tight nodules located in the muscles. Thought to occur from lack of blood flow (ischemia) and can radiate pain to other parts of the body.

Vipassana: A type of meditation characterized by insight into the true nature of all things.

Vitalism: A philosophy characterized by the existence of a life force in all living things.

INDEX

To Write to the Author

If you wish to contact the author or would like more information about this book, please write to the author in care of Llewellyn Worldwide and we will forward your request. Both the author and publisher appreciate hearing from you and learning of your enjoyment of this book and how it has helped you. Llewellyn Worldwide cannot guarantee that every letter written to the author can be answered, but all will be forwarded. Please write to:

Dr. Bruce Forciea
℅ Llewellyn Worldwide
2143 Wooddale Drive, Dept. 978-0-7387-1077-8
Woodbury, MN 55125-2989, U.S.A.

Please enclose a self-addressed stamped envelope for reply, or $1.00 to cover costs. If outside the U.S.A., enclose international postal reply coupon.